The Education of Children and Young People in State Care

T0264894

Young people who leave care with few or no educational qualifications are at very high risk of social exclusion in adulthood. Yet in the past their education has attracted little attention from researchers or professionals. Studies by the editors and contributors to this volume show that the educational standards attained by young people in care fall progressively behind those of their peers living with their own families. This research-based book looks at the educational experiences of children and youths in nine different European countries and Canada. It identifies the obstacles that prevent them from realising their aspirations and discusses ways of improving their opportunities.

How can countries with different traditions, welfare regimes and administrative systems learn from each other? What needs to be done at national, local and individual levels to give children in care equal chances with those living with their families? At present a child in public care is five times less likely to go to university than others. How can teachers, social workers and carers better support their educational attainment, and enable more of them to succeed and progress to tertiary education?

This book was originally published as a special issue of the *European Journal of Social Work*.

Sonia Jackson is an Emeritus Professor at University College London (UCL) Institute of Education, London, UK. She has published over 80 books and articles on children in out-of-home care. As a Psychologist and Social Worker, she first drew attention to the neglect of their education in the 1980s and has continued to research and highlight the issue in many different countries.

Ingrid Höjer is a Professor in the Department of Social Work at the University of Göteborg, Sweden, and has directed many research projects on children and young people in foster care.

The Education of Children and Young People in State Care

Edited by
Sonia Jackson and Ingrid Höjer

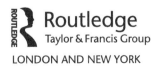
Routledge
Taylor & Francis Group

LONDON AND NEW YORK

First published 2016 by Routledge

2 Park Square, Milton Park, Abingdon, Oxon OX14 4RN
711 Third Avenue, New York, NY 10017, USA

Routledge is an imprint of the Taylor & Francis Group, an informa business

First issued in paperback 2017

British Library Cataloguing in Publication Data
A catalogue record for this book is available from the British Library

ISBN 13: 978-1-138-93486-3 (hbk)
ISBN 13: 978-1-138-09912-8 (pbk)

Typeset in Minion
by RefineCatch Limited, Bungay, Suffolk

Publisher's Note
The publisher accepts responsibility for any inconsistencies that may have
arisen during the conversion of this book from journal articles to book chapters,
namely the possible inclusion of journal terminology.

Disclaimer
Every effort has been made to contact copyright holders for their permission to
reprint material in this book. The publishers would be grateful to hear from any
copyright holder who is not here acknowledged and will undertake to rectify
any errors or omissions in future editions of this book.

Contents

CONTENTS

Citation Information

The chapters in this book were originally published in the *European Journal of Social Work*, volume 16, issue 1 (February 2013). When citing this material, please use the original page numbering for each article, as follows:

Editorial
Prioritising education for children looked after away from home
Sonia Jackson & Ingrid Höjer
European Journal of Social Work, volume 16, issue 1 (February 2013) pp. 1–5

Chapter 1
Delayed educational pathways and risk of social exclusion: the case of young people from public care in Spain
Carme Montserrat, Ferran Casas & Sara Malo
European Journal of Social Work, volume 16, issue 1 (February 2013) pp. 6–21

Chapter 2
School as an opportunity and resilience factor for young people placed in care
Ingrid Höjer & Helena Johansson
European Journal of Social Work, volume 16, issue 1 (February 2013) pp. 22–36

Chapter 3
The importance of social relationships for young people from a public care background
Inge M. Bryderup & Marlene Q. Trentel
European Journal of Social Work, volume 16, issue 1 (February 2013) pp. 37–54

Chapter 4
Enabling young people with a care background to stay in education in Hungary: accommodation with conditions and support
Andrea Rácz & Márta Korintus
European Journal of Social Work, volume 16, issue 1 (February 2013) pp. 55–69

Chapter 5

Placement, protective and risk factors in the educational success of young people in care: cross-sectional and longitudinal analyses
Robert J. Flynn, Nicholas G. Tessier & Daniel Coulombe
European Journal of Social Work, volume 16, issue 1 (February 2013) pp. 70–87

Chapter 6

Addressing low attainment of children in public care: the Scottish experience
Graham Connelly & Judy Furnivall
European Journal of Social Work, volume 16, issue 1 (February 2013) pp. 88–104

Chapter 7

The managerialist turn and the education of young offenders in state care
Tiago Neves
European Journal of Social Work, volume 16, issue 1 (February 2013) pp. 105–119

Chapter 8

Action competence—a new trial aimed at social innovation in residential homes?
Niels Rosendal Jensen
European Journal of Social Work, volume 16, issue 1 (February 2013) pp. 120–136

Chapter 9

The relevance and experience of education from the perspective of Croatian youth in-care
Branka Sladović Franz & Vanja Branica
European Journal of Social Work, volume 16, issue 1 (February 2013) pp. 137–152

For any permission-related enquiries please visit:
http://www.tandfonline.com/page/help/permissions

Notes on Contributors

Vanja Branica is an Assistant Professor in the Department of Social Work at the University of Zagreb, Croatia.

Inge M. Bryderup is a Professor in the Department of Sociology and Social Work at the University of Aalborg, Denmark.

Ferran Casas is Senior Professor of Social Psychology in the Faculty of Education and Psychology at the University of Girona, Spain. His main topics of research are well-being and quality of life, children's rights, adolescents and audio-visual media, families' quality of life in city environments and intergenerational relationships.

Graham Connelly is a Senior Lecturer in the School of Social Work and Social Policy at the University of Strathclyde, Glasgow, UK. He leads the improving educational outcomes of looked after children programme in CELCIS – the Centre for Excellence for Looked After Children in Scotland.

Daniel Coulombe recently retired from his position as an Associate Professor in the School of Psychology at the University of Ottawa, Canada.

Robert J. Flynn is an Emeritus Professor in the School of Psychology and a Senior Researcher at the Centre for Research on Educational and Community Service at the University of Ottawa, Canada.

Judy Furnivall is a Consultancy Lead in CELCIS – the Centre for Excellence for Looked After Children in Scotland, at the University of Strathclyde, Glasgow, UK.

Ingrid Höjer is a Professor in the Department of Social Work at the University of Göteborg, Sweden, and has directed many research projects on children and young people in foster care.

Sonia Jackson is an Emeritus Professor at University College London (UCL) Institute of Education, London, UK. She has published over 80 books and articles on children in out-of-home care. As a Psychologist and Social Worker, she first drew attention to the neglect of their education in the 1980s and has continued to research and highlight the issue in many different countries.

Niels Rosendal Jensen is an Associate Professor in the Research Programme in Social Pedagogy, Inclusive Education, Professionalism and Leadership in the Department of Education at Aarhus University, Denmark.

Helena Johansson is a doctoral student in the Department of Mathematical Sciences at the University of Göteborg, Sweden.

Márta Korintus is the Director of Research at the National Institute for Family and Social Policy in Hungary. She has been involved in work concerning services for children under the age of 3 for more than twenty years.

Sara Malo is tenured Assistant Professor at the University of Girona and a Researcher in the Quality of Life Research Institute (IRQV), Spain.

Carme Montserrat is tenured Assistant Professor at the University of Girona and a Researcher in the Quality of Life Research Institute (IRQV), Spain.

Tiago Neves is Assistant Professor in the Faculty of Psychology and Education at the Universidade do Porto and a Researcher at the Centro de Investigação e Intervenção Educativas, Portugal.

Andrea Rácz is an Adjunct in the Department of Sociology and Social Policy at the University of Debrecen, Hungary.

Branka Sladović Franz is a Researcher in the Department of Social Work at the University of Zagreb, Croatia.

Nicholas G. Tessier is a recent graduate of the PhD programme in Clinical Psychology in the School of Psychology at the University of Ottawa, Canada.

Marlene Q. Trentel is a Research Assistant in the Danish School of Education at the University of Aarhus, Denmark.

INTRODUCTION

Prioritising education for children looked after away from home

The idea for this special issue of the journal arose from a cross-national research project funded under the European Union Seventh Framework Program on Youth and Social Inclusion. The five-country project, known by the acronym YiPPEE (young people in public care—pathways to education in Europe), focused on the post-compulsory education of young men and women who had been looked after away from home as children, and was coordinated by the England team based at the University of London Institute of Education (Jackson & Cameron, 2011). The five countries forming the YiPPEE partnership were chosen to represent different welfare regimes, and the hypothesis was that these would significantly differentiate the educational opportunities and outcomes of children and young people in care, although this was only partly borne out by the results. Four of the papers in this issue of EJSW are based on research by the YiPPEE national teams. The England findings are reported elsewhere (Cameron et al., 2012; Jackson & Cameron, 2012) and in two forthcoming books.

Each of the five countries reviewed the literature in their own language and in English, and these reviews formed a consolidated international overview (Höjer, et al., 2008), which showed that the education of children in care had attracted almost no attention in any country other than the UK, and the educational pathways of children in care beyond legally obligatory school attendance were virtually unknown. This was not altogether a surprise. As long ago as 1983, the gap between care and education systems was identified as the main reason for the neglect of education in the lives of children separated from their families (Jackson, 1987). This division persists, though slightly modified in England by new administrative arrangements bringing social care and education together in Departments of Children's Services (Jackson, 2010), and is clearly reflected in the paucity of academic articles concerned with the school experience and educational attainment of children and young people in public care.

Why does this matter? First, school is of central importance in the everyday life of all children. A child who is unhappy or isolated in the school community is unlikely to make good progress in learning or social development. School difficulties are reflected in placement problems and have been shown, for example by research

1

in Scotland, to be a frequent factor in placement breakdown (Francis, 2000). Conversely, instability of placement, as many of the papers in this issue demonstrate, is a major obstacle to achievement for most children in care. But the second reason is the importance of educational attainment for future life chances. There is a huge body of research showing the close association of positive and negative life course outcomes with the highest level of educational qualification achieved (Simon & Owen, 2006). Children in care have to overcome acute biographical disadvantage if they are to achieve successful integration into adult society. Without educational qualifications giving them access to employment, and lacking the family support available to other young people, they are at very high risk of all the ills associated with social exclusion: welfare dependency, homelessness, drug and alcohol addiction, early parenthood, conflictual relationships, extreme poverty, stigmatisation and crime.

Educational research since the end of the Second World War has shown that home background is a critical factor in school attainment, especially the interest and expectations shown by parents in their children's progress. Yet this has never been high on the social work agenda, for example in approval of foster parents, decisions about placement, choice of school, support for learning difficulties and compensation for missed attendance. By contrast, EU social policy lays great emphasis on raising the educational level of the whole population, reducing early leaving (which includes failing to progress into upper secondary education) and ensuring that all young people are better educated than their parents (European Commission, 2012). This is especially important for those who grow up or spend an extended period in care. The YiPPEE research found that in all partner countries the 170 young people who took part in the in-depth phase of the study came from very similar families, a high proportion of which could be characterised as socially excluded. By the time they reached adolescence almost all had parents who were separated or divorced. Abuse and neglect, domestic violence, alcoholism and drug addiction featured in most of the research participants' accounts. They themselves recognised that education is the best, if not the only, means by which they can hope to avoid repeating the dysfunctional life patterns of their birth families.

In some countries, notably Sweden, the majority of children in care do cross the first hurdle, the examination at the end of compulsory schooling, but after that they face increasing obstacles to accessing higher levels of education. In the UK fewer than one in five even get to first base. The European target of 40% of the whole youth population accessing tertiary education looks far out of reach for those in care. The YiPPEE studies found that only between 3 and 13% of young people in care entered university even in countries with more generous welfare regimes. The social work profession must accept some of the responsibility for the gross discrepancy in educational opportunity between children in care and others. A consistent finding noted in the YiPPEE literature review, as well as in several of the following papers, is that most social workers take only a cursory interest in school experience or educational attainment and generally attribute poor progress to individual characteristics of children rather than to weaknesses in the system. In research based on first-hand accounts by young people themselves, it is striking how few attribute success to support from social workers.

We are pleased to be able to include in this special issue papers from seven different European countries, representing a range of different welfare regimes, as well as one from Canada. North American studies can often draw on larger samples and provide valuable quantitative evidence to support (or challenge) conclusions of smaller scale and qualitative research. Robert Flynn, Nicholas Tessier and Daniel Coulombe report on a study in Ontario, where a basic model of educational success drawing on resilience theory was tested on a sample of 1106 young people in care.

Among the European papers resilience is also a dominant theme. The paper from Sweden, by Ingrid Höjer and Helena Johansson, suggests that school is an underrated resource for some young people at risk, as well as those in care. School may constitute a place of structure and safety in contrast to a more chaotic and problematic situation at home or in placement. They found that school also provided access to social capital, and a sense of 'normality', a place where young people from adverse circumstances could see friends and meet interested and committed adults. Inge Bryderup and Marlene Trentel, discussing findings from the YiPPEE study in Denmark, point to the enduring influence of adverse family backgrounds and propose a typology of young people in care relating a variety of characteristics to their educational progress or lack of it. A second paper from Denmark by Niels Rosendal Jensen discusses an innovative scheme aiming to introduce evidence-based practice into residential homes and put much more emphasis on education and social inclusion. Changing institutional culture is notoriously difficult to do but this carefully planned project met with considerable success. In the Spanish context, Carme Montserrat, Ferran Casas and Sara Malo show that young people in public care frequently experience delay in their educational pathways and need longer to reach the same point as their home-based peers. This also applies to those who show educational promise and are highly motivated to continue their studies beyond compulsory schooling. The authors found that professionals in the child protection system did not prioritise education for children and young people placed in public care, and generally had low expectations of their educational achievement. The authors highlight the need for policies to create equality of educational opportunity and reduce the risk of social exclusion for this group of young people.

All the papers illustrate the great importance of structural factors, such as local and national government policies that affect social work and educational practice. There are also strong historical continuities, which have a major impact on children's education and care experiences. Two of the countries included in this issue are in transition from former communist regimes. In relation to children in care this has both positive and negative aspects, as we see from the experience of Hungary and Croatia. Hungary is the only country where upper secondary education (to 18) is technically compulsory, and this clearly benefits children in care. On the other hand, in practice, the quality of education they can access after 14 proved, in the analysis of the YiPPEE findings by Marta Korintus and Andrea Racz, to be very variable and often out of line with their ability. In all countries, opportunities for care leavers are limited by lack of funding and the need for young people to work to support themselves at a much earlier age than their peers.

Graham Connelly and Judy Furnivall provide an account of policy developments within the Scottish legal and educational context, which gives some grounds for optimism. They found considerable infrastructural development, both in the looked-after children sector and in education services, and improvement in outcomes such as school attendance and educational attainment. However, the modest progress that has been made in recent years is extremely vulnerable to changes at the political level. This is only too clear in England, where the strong drive led by the 1997–2010 Labour Government to improve educational outcomes for children in care is currently threatened by savage cuts in local authority funding and the abolition of the Education Maintenance Allowance, a crucial resource in enabling young people to stay in education after 16. Similarly, a conservative swing in Portugal has affected the approach to young people in trouble with the law. Tiago Neves argues that there has been a shift in residential care for offenders from a humanistic perspective, aimed at their social integration, towards a containment regime focused on social control and risk management rather than education and rehabilitation.

We are most grateful to the *European Journal of Social Work* for inviting us to edit a special issue on the education of children in care. Our hope is that this will be only a beginning, and that the lead given by EJSW will stimulate many more submissions to this and other social work journals on a crucial and neglected topic.

References

Cameron, C., Jackson, S., Hauari, H. & Hollingworth, C. (2012) 'Continuing educational participation among children in care in five countries: Some issues of social class', *Journal of Education Policy*, vol. 27, no. 3, pp. 387–399. Available at: http://dx.doi.org/10.1080/02680939.2011.644811

European Commission. (2012) *Youth on the Margins of Society: Policy Review of Research Results*. EU Directorate General for Research and Innovation Socio-Economic Sciences and Humanities EUR25375, Brussels.

Francis, J. (2000) 'Investing in children's futures: Enhancing the educational arrangements of 'looked after' children', *Child and Family Social Work*, vol. 24, no. 3, pp. 241–260.

Höjer, I., Johannson, H., Hill, M., Jackson, S. & Cameron, C. (2008) *State of the Art Consolidated Literature Review: The Educational Pathways of Young People from a Public Care Background in Five EU Countries* (No. WP2), University of Goteborg, Goteborg.

Jackson, S. (1987) *The Education of Children in Care*, University of Bristol Papers in Applied Social Studies, Bristol.

Jackson, S. (2010) 'Reconnecting care and education: from the Children Act 1989 to Care Matters', *Journal of Children's Services*, vol. 5, no 3, pp. 48–60. doi:10.5042/jcs.2010.0550

Jackson, S. & Cameron, C. (2011). *Young People from a Public Care Background: Pathways to Further and Higher Education in Five European Countries*. Final report of the YiPPEE project. Institute of Education, London. Available at: www.ioe.ac.uk/yippee

Jackson, S. & Cameron, C. (2012). 'Leaving care: Looking ahead and aiming higher', *Children and Youth Services Review*, vol. 34, pp. 1107–1114. doi:10.1016/j.childyouth.2012.01.041

Simon, A. & Owen, C. (2006) 'Outcomes for children in care: What do we know?', in *In care and after: A positive perspective*, eds E. Chase, A. Simon & S. Jackson, Routledge, London, pp. 26–43.

Sonia Jackson
Thomas Coram Research Unit Institute of Education
University of London, London, UK

Ingrid Höjer
Department of Social Work, University of Göteborg,
Göteborg, Sweden

Delayed educational pathways and risk of social exclusion: the case of young people from public care in Spain

Retraso en los itinerarios educativos y riesgo de exclusión social: el caso de los jóvenes ex-tutelados en España

Carme Montserrat, Ferran Casas & Sara Malo

It is assumed that education may be one of the key aspects in preventing social exclusion and that children in both residential and family foster care would seem to be at risk of exclusion due to unequal opportunities in compulsory and post-compulsory education, particularly when leaving care. On the basis of findings from a European research project, this article examines the educational pathways in Spain among 18–22 year olds who were in care at 16. The qualitative results presented here were taken from initial and follow-up interviews with young people from a public care background, interviews with care managers and nominated adults—mainly social educators. Results showed that delays in educational pathways were frequent among these young people, even those who showed educational promise and were highly motivated. Factors associated with such delays were related to (1) professionals and managers in the child protection system not prioritising their education; (2) low expectations among adults providing them with support; (3) invisibility within the educational system of the specific support needs of this population and (4) additional difficulties this population encounters in the transition to adulthood. If policies are to be developed to address all of the above factors, it is crucial to assess what urgent changes are required to empower the potential human and social capital of this population, increase equality in their educational opportunities and reduce their high risk of social exclusion.

Se asume que la educación constituye uno de los aspectos clave en la prevención de la exclusión social, y que los niños, tanto en acogimiento residencial y como familiar, parecen estar en riesgo de exclusión debido a la desigualdad de oportunidades educativas, tanto en la escolaridad obligatoria como postobligatoria, y especialmente cuando salen del sistema de protección. A partir de los resultados de un proyecto europeo de investigación, este trabajo examina los itinerarios educativos de una muestra de jóvenes entre los 18–22 años de edad que estaban tutelados a los 16 años. Se presentan los resultados cualitativos, centrados en España, fruto de las entrevistas realizadas a los jóvenes, los profesionales y los adultos de referencia—principalmente educadores sociales. Estos resultados muestran que los retrasos en los itinerarios educativos son frecuentes entre estos jóvenes, incluso en aquellos que presentan capacidad y alta motivación para seguir estudiando. Los factores asociados con los retrasos están relacionados con (1) la poca prioridad que dan a la escolaridad los profesionales y directivos en el sistema de protección a la infancia, (2) las bajas expectativas que los adultos tienen en los niños y adolescentes tutelados, (3) la invisibilidad en el sistema educativo de las necesidades específicas de apoyo que tiene esta población, y (4) las dificultades adicionales que estos jóvenes encuentran en su transición hacia la edad adulta. Para el desarrollo de políticas que tengan en cuenta estos factores obstaculizadores, es crucial empezar a valorar qué cambios deben implementarse con urgencia de cara a potenciar el capital humano y social de esta población, aumentar la igualdad en sus oportunidades educativas y reducir el alto riesgo de exclusión social.

Introduction

We know very little about the situation of children and adolescents in the Spanish protection system when it comes to their schooling. We know even less about the educational pathways these young people follow after leaving the protection system, and almost nothing about the factors underlying this population subgroup's dropping out of school and low academic achievements.

Jackson (2010a) points out how the issue of school was ignored for decades by most European protection (child welfare) systems. In Spain, the principle of normalisation applied (Casas, 1998) from the 1980s onwards led to the disappearance of macro-institutions in the transition to democracy, resulting in children receiving their education at state schools or state-subsidised private schools, away from the residential home. Perhaps a further step—and the most important one—was still missing, however, providing the education system with tools to promote the integration of these children so that taking schooling outside the residential home would not mean the protection system washing its hands of responsibility in this area. In fact, it is common to hear professionals in the protection system attributing sole responsibility to the school when it comes to education, and the schools attributing sole responsibility to the protection services for meeting the specific educational needs of these young people.

The lack of published data when it comes to educational results, referred to by some authors as 'statistical invisibility' (Casas, 1998; Casas & Montserrat, 2009), has contributed to keeping this reality hidden and also, therefore, to neither side implementing programmes due to lack of awareness of the 'problem'.

Data from the UK (Cameron *et al.*, 2011) show that the percentage of young people in the protection system who complete secondary education is only 41.2%, compared to 90.5% of the general population.

In Catalonia (Montserrat, Casas, *et al.*, 2010), the rate for those students passing secondary education at 15 is 69.4% among the general population, compared to 31.7% of the care population (Table 1), significant differences being observed between those at a residential home and those in non-kinship foster care and kinship foster care. Difficulties at school, both social and academic, are also highlighted in other Spanish studies (Del Valle *et al.*, 2009; Martín *et al.*, 2008), particularly for not only those in residential care, but also those in foster care.

Data are available from Denmark (Bryderup *et al.*, 2010) for not only the level of education achieved by young people between the ages of 18 and 22 who have left care, but also their level of education when aged between 27 and 30; post-compulsory upper secondary education (equivalent to *Bachillerato* or initial vocational training courses) was completed by only 2.5% in the 18–22 age range and 30.8% in the 27–30 age range, compared to 37.6 and 46.1% of the general population. With regard to further education, only 7.3% of young people aged 27–30 who had passed through the protection system had completed it, compared to 34.7% of the general population.

Table 1.   Percentages of Students Passing Secondary Education at 15

	General population	Care population ($n = 265$)		
		Residential home	Kinship family	Non-kinship family
Percentages of students passing secondary education at 15	69.4	23.4	45.5	40.0
			31.7	

Note: 2009–2010 school year.

In Sweden (Hojer & Johansson, 2010), 38% of young people leaving care completed post-compulsory upper secondary education, compared to 85% of the general population.

There has been a recent suspicion that these isolated data for different countries may prove to be very similar if obtained for all countries. Studies show that among all of the social groups identified, young people leaving care are most likely to experience teenage pregnancy, health problems and delinquency (Jackson, 2010b), all situations associated with a lack of employment and dependency on the welfare services. The study Evaluation of Formal Training (2001–2008) compiled by the Higher Council for the Evaluation of Education in Catalonia (2010) suggests that labour market integration for Vocational Training graduates (five years after finishing their studies) is between 11 and 20% higher than for those who did not continue their studies; income is also between 23 and 28% higher.

It is vital to identify the factors influencing why young people entering the care system after significantly falling behind at school not only do not manage to compensate for their delays or deficits, but why these often become worse as they pass through the system (O'Sullivan & Westerman, 2007; Casas *et al.*, 2010).

Studies by Stein and Munro (2008), and others conducted in Spain by Montserrat and Casas (2010), Del Valle *et al.* (2003) and García Barriocanal *et al.* (2007), highlight those factors which facilitate and hinder social integration for these young people when they leave the system and continue with their process of independence. The stability they enjoyed in the protection system, support services for those leaving care, the involvement of a tutor and a social support network, mainly comprising friends, present themselves as the most facilitating factors. Labelling and stigmatisation processes (Casas *et al.*, 2000), as well as low expectations of them, which among the general population may even lead to them being considered potential offenders or abusers, or in the best case scenario, only being expected to become unqualified workers, are the factors which pose an obstacle to their social integration.

In their studies into foster care, Colton *et al.* (2004) point out that for young people, entering the protection system means beginning to participate in a school drop-out culture. According to these authors, school is one of the aspects of their lives in which it is most essential to maintain continuity in the relationship with teachers and friends, class attendance, not falling behind academically and so on, issues which must be taken more into account by social and child protection services. A further key issue is to study and assess the quality of care received by foster children, in order to determine how this affects their well-being. Most studies indicate that the childcare population suffer higher rates of emotional, social, behavioural and school problems than the general population (Rutter, 2000). Various authors agree in considering school to be one of the most relevant aspects in the present and future well-being and quality of life among those who have been in the protection system (Shlonsky & Berrick, 2001; Hunt, 2003).

The data presented here, taken from a sample in Catalonia, were collected within the context of a European research project (YIPPEE) aimed at taking a more in-depth look at which factors facilitate or hinder young people leaving care from continuing in post-compulsory and further education, in addition to their academic performance (Casas *et al.*, 2010).

Much of the theory is taken from approaches that endorse studying the views of the social agents involved in order to understand complex social situations, within on one hand a broader framework of studies into quality of life (Casas, 1998). On the other hand, there is the ecological perspective of studies into abuse (Bronfenbrenner, 1979/1987) that explain the coexistence of a variety of factors intervening at different systemic levels of the process.

Method

Participants

The qualitative study was carried out using three samples: professionals from the social welfare services ($n = 13$), young people leaving care ($n = 35$ in the first round, repeating the interview with 28 of them one year later) and adults nominated by these young people ($n = 20$). A total of 96 interviews were conducted.

We first used an ad hoc sample of key informants, all of them managers of welfare services from the Catalan support service for young people leaving care (Àrea de Suport als Joves Tutelats i Extutelats [ASJTET], 2010), interdisciplinary child protection teams (EAIA) and the local Social Services.

The criteria for selecting the sample of young people leaving care were the same as those used in the European project: 35 young people from each country, aged between 19 and 21, who had been in the protection system for a minimum of one year, who had been in it at the age of 16 and who at that age had showed the ability and motivation to continue into post-compulsory education. In this country, we decided that this would equate to having successfully graduated from secondary school at 16, having begun vocational training or upper secondary education and showing motivation to participate in further education. Of this sample of young people leaving care, 28 were interviewed again one year later (2009).

We asked the young people interviewed to nominate an adult who had given them a special or key support during their schooling. A total of 20 interviews were completed with these nominated people, of whom 17 were social educators at the residential homes, 2 child protection service professionals and 1 a foster family member.

Instruments

In order to collect the data we designed:

- One initial questionnaire aimed at the young people, to compile basic personal information.
- One semi-structured interview aimed at the welfare services professionals.

- One in-depth interview, with an autobiographical format, aimed at the young people leaving care (first round).
- One semi-structured follow-up interview aimed at the same young people (second round), conducted 12 months later.
- One semi-structured interview aimed at the adults nominated by the young people.

Procedure

Authorisation was requested and obtained from the Catalan government to conduct the research, including an agreement to respect the current privacy and confidentiality regulations for the aforementioned data. All interviews were conducted with the free and informed consent of participants, who were notified of their right to not respond to any questions they deemed inappropriate and withdraw from the study at any time without reason.

Data Analysis

After all of the interviews had been transcribed, we proceeded with the analysis of the data, following the stages proposed by Bardin (2002), and using version 8.0 of the qualitative data analysis programme NVivo. The following stages were followed: pre-analysis, exploring the material and results processing. Following this sequence, we then read the transcripts of the interviews for the first time in order to familiarise ourselves with the material and establish operative criteria for the analysis. In the second stage of exploring the material we opted to analyse the content by categories. Successive and independent readings of the transcripts by various members of the research team led to its subsequent review.

Characteristics of the Sample of Young People

In order to contextualise the results, we include here a description of the characteristics of the young people interviewed, data taken from a questionnaire administered before the in-depth interview. Most of them (65.7%) had been in residential homes. By gender, 24 of the young people interviewed were female (68.6%), which means that they were over-represented if compared with the percentage for the care population in Spain, which has more young men than young women. However, this bias is due to the fact that sampling included only those 'having successfully graduated from secondary school at 16', this being achieved more often among girls than among boys. As much as 74.3% of the sample had Spanish nationality and 22.8% had a temporary residence permit linked to a work contract. By country of origin, 12 (34.3%) were born outside Spain, of whom 5 (14.3%) were unaccompanied foreign minors, all male and African; 71.4% of the young people interviewed lived in the province of Barcelona, and their geographical distribution being very similar to that of young people of the same age among the general population (71.8%).

In the case of over half of the young people, one or both parents had died or their whereabouts were unknown. Most had suffered situations of abuse or neglect during their childhood. In the cases where they still had a relationship with their parents, this was usually not very steady; the young person visited them or was visited by them, but they did not represent any type of support for the young person. All except four of them had siblings and one-third of the young people assumed some kind of responsibility towards their younger siblings. Some of them had a partner, but none had children. Half of them lived in accommodation for care leavers. Those who had been in foster families continued to live with them, and 37% lived independently. None of them lived with their birth parents. Generally speaking, they said they were in good health, although three were undergoing psychiatric treatment.

In the first interview (aged between 18 and 21), one-fifth of the sample had abandoned their studies and were working or looking for work. Half were working full-time, and some had managed to combine work and study. The type of work they did was mainly non-qualified. With regard to the highest level of study they had achieved, 5 were at university at the time of the interview, 12 had begun an advanced vocational training course (CFGS), of whom 2 had finished it, 5 had reached upper secondary education, with 2 of them obtaining the qualification, 10 had begun an intermediate vocational training course (CFGM), 7 of whom had obtained the corresponding qualification, 1 had the qualification for completing compulsory secondary education and 2 had the attendance certificate. More females and Spanish nationals were found at the higher levels.

In the initial questionnaire they were asked to give a score from 0 to 10 (from completely dissatisfied to completely satisfied) for their satisfaction with different areas relating to education and their overall life. The results show an average overall life satisfaction of 7.76 (SD = 1.84), a similar score to that obtained by young people in the general population in Catalonia. Their satisfaction is also quite high for the other life domains, the lowest being related to academic results ($M = 6.71$, SD = 1.51).

However, despite the fact that 90% of the young people in our sample graduated from secondary school at the expected age (16) and were motivated and satisfied with their studies, their post-compulsory education became progressively more delayed and ultimately indefinite, to the extent that 78% of those taking an advanced vocational training course did so later than usual. What is more, 20% were no longer studying at the time of the first interview.

By comparing the characteristics displayed by the 35 young people interviewed and the overall in-care population in Catalonia, we could observe that in our sample there were (1) no differences regarding the type of abuse experienced, (2) a higher percentage of young women and a lower proportion of early school leavers, possibly explained by the selection criterion of showing educational promise, (3) an over-representation of young people who have been in a residential home, possibly due to more contact facilities obtained from post-care services and (4) a much lower percentage of young people returning to their birth family upon reaching adulthood.

Results

The data indicated that the academic results of the care population were far below than those of the general population, even after having spent years in the protection system under professional supervision. Only a minority of young people in the system continued studying, and even those who showed the ability and motivation to continue into post-compulsory and further education encountered serious difficulties in doing so; they generally experienced delays and some abandoned their attempts. It is of vital importance to obtain and understand their view of this in order to identify the barriers they come up against. The views of welfare services professionals have also contributed to our understanding in this area.

Which factors have been identified that may facilitate or hinder this complex process of school and social integration for the protection system population? Contributions from the aforementioned social agents point mainly to the following.

Professionals and Managers in the Child Protection System Not Prioritising the Education of This Population

The young people were aware of the extent to which, at the residential home or in the foster family, their schooling was prioritised and specifically organised (or not). Their unanimous view was that it was easier to study when with a foster family than at a home. The young people and professionals referred to the difficulties of studying at certain homes, whilst also recognising the effort made by some social educators in homes to facilitate studying.

Those who lived in residential homes particularly complained about constant changes in social educators and the fact that they worked in shifts. They regarded this as a disadvantage when it came to sharing their problems with them, including school problems. Living with a foster family was more positive in this respect. The social educators interviewed agreed that there are too many changes in personnel.

Furthermore, it is difficult to believe that schooling is being prioritised if stability in the foster placement is not prioritised at the same time. The constant changes of residence and key adults in the protection system clearly have a negative impact on their schooling, leading to changes of school and making it difficult for them to keep up with schoolwork, as well as losing friends, an issue which receives strong emphasis from the young people interviewed.

A point of view defended particularly strongly by the young people interviewed was the importance of their opinion being heard and taken into account. They believed it particularly important that they took part in decisions that affect their lives, lamenting that this was unfortunately not a widespread practice in the protection system.

Girl aged 19:

> I said to them 'OK, if I go to a home it has to be under the condition that I can leave it, that it is close to my home so I can see my family, and that they let me go to the same school'.

Low Expectations Among Adults Providing Them with Support

The professionals interviewed had very low expectations when it came to the young people in the protection system. This was apparent to the young people themselves, and they also felt the weight of being labelled by society as a person 'with problems', 'a delinquent' or 'future abuser', whether in the media, their community, at school, or even in the protection system itself.

Social services professionals considered it difficult to find pathways for them in formal education. The young people clearly perceived the difference between those social educators who did not expect much when it came to their education and those who encouraged them to have higher aspirations.

The latter transmitted the value of education, and the young people interviewed generally viewed education as being key to leaving behind their difficult social situation. This was also true of the professionals, who stated that getting educated can help them to become more valued in life, have a choice of job and improve their economic situation. However, the young people did not see clear actions accompanying these words. The professionals admitted that enough progress had not been made in this respect.

Most of the young people and social educators believed that the former were less likely to abandon their studies if social educators at the residential homes provided them with constant help and closely monitored their situation at school (homework and exam preparation, meetings with the school tutor, participation in school and extra-curricular activities, finding them a private tutor, etc.)

Young man aged 19:

> It's something I still have to do ... find that teacher and ..., thank her, more than anything ... for pressuring me to pass and make the effort. (...) this teacher in primary school who made me see that I had to study to ... because my life was already difficult, and I had to study because if I didn't it would become much more difficult, so I knew that the key was to study. To get to university.

Invisibility Within the Educational System of the Specific Support Needs
of This Population Deriving from Family Circumstances, Trauma
or Other Situations

There are no regular statistics, nor even isolated data to reflect the academic situation of these children in Spain (those collected during this study being the first), and neither has any programme been identified for this population within the education system. This was unanimously corroborated by the professionals interviewed and was also the perception of the young people. These were children who changed schools often, lost their friends and suffered delays in their academic progress. Some were not there long enough for the teachers to get to know them, assess their needs and implement some means of support.

Girl aged 21:

> I actually learnt to read in Year 4. Because changing from school to school . . . and I
> didn't even go to a special class or anything to learn to read . . . I tricked the teachers
> a lot, because . . . I learnt the books by heart, I told my brother to read them to me,
> and I learnt them by memory. (. . .) when they said: read (. . .) I recited what I had
> learnt. Until one day, because I'm dyslexic, one day, when I reached (. . .) year 4 or 5
> my maths teacher, he realised I was dyslexic.

When the school is sensitive, it welcomes children and young people who have passed
through the protection system, and adapts to their specific situation. For example, it
recognises that the reason that they have fallen behind academically is due to previous
disruption, changes of placement and school and gaps in attendance. Often they join
the school halfway through the school year, with people who are not part of their
family and have to adjust to a different structure from that of a residential home. The
welfare services professionals were very critical of the lack of knowledge and
involvement of some schools, and some social educators stated that it is fundamental
for the school to want and be able to help these young people to progress. They
themselves related both good and bad practices:

Young man aged 19:

> I have always had a good relationship with teachers, no problem. And I have always
> been able to trust them so that I could explain the situation, and they also helped
> me a little. But they've never gone out of their way to help me, eh!(. . .). I've had to
> work as hard as the others but they've helped me . . . to organise myself better and
> all that, and to trust them.

His social educator at the home:

> He had a mentor, and the psychologist and the head of studies helped him a lot.
> School helped him a lot. It was they who found out about his situation and
> informed the Social Services; at the beginning they were very involved.

Additional Difficulties This Population Encounters in the Transition to Adulthood Compared with Those Encountered by an Average Young Person in the Country

In Catalonia, social services professionals and social educators can turn to the post-
care service to help those young people who ask for support and agree to the
conditions of the service. A large proportion of them were grateful for the support
that had allowed them to go to care leaver accommodation, receive a grant or a
private tutor. The uncertainty they felt when reaching the age of 18 means taking
decisions based on immediate priorities. This was why the young people and
professionals interviewed highlight the importance of young people leaving care
being able to count on support services such as care leaver accommodation or
student residences, student grants and personal support for those who need it, in
order to alleviate the fear and insecurity arising from reaching legal adulthood

without family support. This was particularly the case if they wished to study, as without this support it is very difficult to continue studying.

All of the professionals interviewed valued short-term study options and early incorporation into the labour market for young people from the protection system, even when the young person had the motivation and ability to choose a pathway in further education. The young people interviewed were aware of this tendency and some of them felt it was completely unfair.

Her social educator at the home:

> When she told us she wanted to do general upper secondary education and go to university we did tell her to keep her feet on the ground. We told her: 'you're going to leave here, who's going to pay for your studies? How are you going to manage it? (...) if you don't want to go back to your family, you need to earn money to have a flat' (...) we talked to her and I saw the need for her to do some vocational training and work.

Discussion

The young people find themselves in the paradoxical situation of being told that studying is important, but the advice and actions of professionals conveying the opposite. On the contrary, they are advised to find work as soon as possible, the physical conditions and specific support to be able to study is missing at some homes and they face instability both inside the homes and in changing homes. The question is, is schooling really prioritised and the value of education really transmitted? The professionals interviewed accept that urgent improvements are required in this respect. Authors such as Jackson (2010a) have been highlighting this deficiency for years.

Stability in their care placements is one of the factors that is gradually becoming more accepted as essential to the well-being of this population (Del Valle *et al.*, 2003; Sinclair *et al.*, 2007; Stein & Munro, 2008). Despite this, it is still common to find continuous changes in most of the systems (Jackson & Sachdev, 2001; Colton *et al.*, 2004). Such instability leads on many occasions to changes of school and is harmful on different levels: falling behind academically, losing friends and a lesser likelihood that the school will detect specific needs and develop a corresponding programme. Research that has awarded credibility to the version given by the children themselves illustrates how they suffer in this respect. Ward *et al.* (2005) highlight the negative perception the children have of a change in foster care, how this affects their whole personal, family and school life, whilst entailing a change of doctor and losing belongings.

In Spain, children often suffer changes of residential home due to age, behaviour or the home closing down, but they also suffer due to changes of tutor in the home, changes of personnel due to shift work or high staff turnover. Kinship foster care provides greater stability (Farmer & Moyers, 2008; Montserrat, 2008), as was also observed in this study. Authors such as Del Valle and García Barriocanal find instability in itself to be more harmful than the number of years spent in the system. These results also agree with those found by Montserrat, González, *et al.* (2010). At homes with low numbers, more trusting relationships can be established with the social educator (Del Valle & Casas, 2002) than at larger homes, an aspect also emphasised by some of the young people interviewed and their social educators.

That said, the influence does not stem simply from a bond with a reference adult or someone who could be considered a 'resilience mentor' (Cyrulnik, 2002), but rather this person must also become involved in their schooling and transmit high expectations regarding their educational pathway. It is important that they help them do their homework or find someone competent to do this for them, and have a close relationship with their schoolteacher which allows them to participate in all school activities. This person needs to tell them they will become good cooks or doctors, that they have the ability to achieve what they want and that they will help them to do so. According to the young people, they need people who do not think that they will follow the same life path as their parents and that they can only end up as unskilled workers; they place great value on a positive outlook. They feel the weight of social labelling and self-fulfilling prophecies (Casas *et al.*, 2000).

Despite this, the high level of overall satisfaction that most of the young people in our sample express regarding their lives is very striking. In general they are resilient and tend to be optimistic about their future, a phenomenon also observed by Montserrat and Casas (2007) and Montserrat, González, *et al.* (2010).

We know the beneficial effects of a positive feeling of belonging, something which is boosted when the group is well regarded socially (Tajfel, 1984), as is the case with students who are academically successful. For young people from the protection system, forming part of a group with these characteristics is key to their integration in the formal education system. Having a group of friends from outside the protection system is a very significant facilitating factor in their social integration (Bravo & Del Valle, 2001), helping them to have a normal environment and daily life (Casas, 1998).

The involvement of the school is fundamental, and this is perhaps where most time should be invested in designing programmes to respond to the needs of these children. It is worth noting that these young people want to be helped, but they do not receive a special treatment. School can constitute an integrating factor in compensating for the labelling they have to bear due to being in the protection system; or conversely, it can be a place where their failure is once again highlighted, thereby contributing to their being doubly labelled, which is difficult to overcome. For example, the education system has programmes for students with disabilities or immigrants. How many programmes do we know that are aimed at the care population?

The issue of listening to the young people themselves also requires urgent improvement, and it is they in particular who alert us to this defect in the protection systems. In respect of this, Colton *et al.* (2004) point out that despite being in foster care, these children still share the same fundamental needs as other children, and wish to be heard on issues that directly affect them (see also the Council of Europe recommendation, 2009), one of which is their experience of school.

The social agents consulted are unanimous in stating that the school guidance these young people receive tends to be directed towards short-term professional training and early labour market insertion. In another study conducted in Girona,

Spain, the young people interviewed also had low-level qualifications and were therefore more susceptible to suffering from instability and a precarious working situation (Montserrat, González, et al., 2010). They also stated that they had received guidance very much focused on labour market insertion in order to leave the residential home already having a job.

A fundamental factor contributing to a favourable independence process (Ward et al., 2006; Stein & Munro, 2008) is being able to count on effective support when they leave the system: personal support, the social educator's involvement in the area of education, housing support, grants or psychological help, depending on the young person in question. In this respect, it is worth highlighting the role played by the post-care service in Catalonia over the last 15 years (2010).

The 35 young people interviewed do not live with their birth family, whilst data from the Youth Secretariat (2008) show that in Catalonia up to the age of 29 more than 50% of young people in the general population live with their parents. This is a very important point for the social inclusion of the population of Catalan care leavers, who cannot depend on parental support and for whom the transition to an independent life generally occurs very quickly, meaning that the majority are forced to find work urgently, resulting in the abandonment of education.

Recommendations

The results obtained lead us to three complementary reflections. On the one hand, the child protection system must adopt a new attitude towards schooling, with formal education occupying a central and prioritised place in the life of young people during residential or family foster care, as well as during the process of leaving the protection system.

On the other hand, the education system must consider these students to be a group with specific educational needs, taking into account their family circumstances and the traumatic experiences suffered during their lives, guaranteeing them a support even after the period of compulsory education.

Finally, the two systems must improve (or initiate) coordination to resolve the serious inequality in educational opportunities for young people in and leaving care, which tends to lead to difficulties in labour market insertion due to their low level of qualifications, and often even a high risk of long-term unemployment and social exclusion. This coordination must bring with it a means of compensating for and overcoming their accumulated academic deficit, rather than aggravating it during their time in the protection system, as we usually see happening in the current situation.

Acknowledgements

The research leading to these results received funds from the European Union's Seventh Framework Programme under grant agreement no. 217297. The research project was undertaken by a team of cross-national researchers from: the Danish School of Education University of Aarhus, Denmark; the Institute for Social Policy and Labour, Hungary; the Research Institute on Quality of Life, University of Girona, Spain; the Department of Social Work and the Department of Education, University of Gothenburg; and the Thomas Coram Research Unit, Institute of Education, University of London, England. All the researchers contributed to the research reported here, but responsibility for this article lies with the authors. The views expressed in this article are those of the authors and not necessarily those of other partners or of the European Union.

References

Àrea de Suport als Joves Tutelats i Extutelats (ASJTET). (2010) *Mèmoria 2009* [Report, 2009], Generalitat de Catalunya, Barcelona.

Bardin, L. (2002) *Análisis de contenido* [*Content analysis*], Akal, Madrid.

Bravo, A. & Del Valle, J. F. (2001) 'Evaluación de la integración social en acogimiento residencial', *Psicothema*, vol. 13, no. 2, pp. 197–204.

Bronfenbrenner, U. (1979/1987) *La ecología del desarrollo humano* [*The Ecology of Human Development*], Paidós, Barcelona.

Bryderup, I. M., Quisgaard Trentel, M. & Kring, T. (2010) 'WP3 & 4 – analysis of quantitative data from Denmark. The YIPPEE Project', [Online] Available at: http://tcru.ioe.ac.uk/yippee

Cameron, C., Hollingworth, K. & Jackson, S. (ed.) (2011) 'Secondary analysis of national statistics on educational participation. The YIPPEE Project', [Online] Available at: http://tcru.ioe.ac.uk/yippee

Casas, F. (1998) *Infancia: Perspectivas psicosociales* [*Childhood: Psychosocial Approach*], Paidós, Barcelona.

Casas, F., Cornejo, J. M., Colton, M. & Scholte, E. (2000) 'Perceptions of stigmatization and satisfaction with services received, among users of social welfare services for the child and family in 3 European regions', *Social Indicators Research*, vol. 51, pp. 287–309.

Casas, F. & Montserrat, C. (2009) 'Sistema educativo e igualdad de oportunidades entre los jóvenes tutelados: estudios recientes en el Reino Unido [*Educational system and equal opportunities for young people in care: Recent studies in the UK*]', *Psicothema*, vol. 21, no. 4, pp. 543–547.

Casas, F., Montserrat, C. & Malo, S. (2010) 'Young people from a public care background pathways to education in Spain. The case study report. The YIPPEE project', [Online] Available at: http://tcru.ioe.ac.uk/yippee

Colton, M., Pithouse, A., Roberts, S. & Ward, H. (2004) *What Works in Practice: A Review of Research Evidence*, National Assembly for Wales, Cardiff.

Consejo de Europa (Council of Europe recommendation). (2009) *Una estrategia integral contra la violencia (Guía)* [*Guidelines on integrated national strategies for the protection of children from violence*], [Online] Available at: www.coe.int/children

Consejo Superior de Evaluación de Cataluña (Higher Council for the Evaluation of Education in Catalonia). (2010) *L'Avaluació de la Formació Reglada (2001–2008)* [*The assessment of formal Education, (2001–2008)*], Generalitat de Catalunya, Barcelona.

Cyrulnik, B. (2002) *Los patitos feos. La resiliencia: una infancia infeliz no determina la vida* [*The Ugly Ducks*], Gedisa, Barcelona.

Del Valle, J., Álvarez, E. & Bravo, A. (2003) 'Evaluación de resultados a largo plazo en acogimiento residencial de protección a la infancia', *Infancia y Aprendizaje*, vol. 26, no. 2, pp. 235–249.

Del Valle, J. F. & Casas, F. (2002) 'Child residential care in the Spanish social protection system', *International Journal of Child & Family Welfare*, vol. 5, no. 3, pp. 112–128.

Del Valle, J. F., López, M., Montserrat, C. & Bravo, A. (2009) 'Twenty years of foster care in Spain: profiles, patterns and outcomes', *Children and Youth Services Review*, vol. 31, pp. 847–853.

Farmer, E. & Moyers, S. (2008) *Kinship Care*, JKP, London.

García Barriocanal, C., Imaña, A. & de la Herrán, A. (2007) *El acogimiento residencial como medida de protección al menor [Residential care within the child protection system]*, Defensor del Menor en la Comunidad de Madrid, Madrid.

Hojer, I. & Johansson, H. (2010) 'WP3 – analysis of quantitative data from Sweden. The YIPPEE Project', [Online] Available at: http://tcru.ioe.ac.uk/yippee

Hunt, J. (2003) 'Family and friends carers', *Scoping paper prepared for the Department of Health*, London, DoH.

Jackson, S. (2010a) 'Reconnecting care and education', *Journal of Children's Services*, vol. 5, no. 3, pp. 48–59.

Jackson, S. (2010b) 'Education for social inclusion. Can we change the future for children in care? An inaugural professorial lecture by Sonia Jackson', [Online] Available at: www.ioe.ac.uk/publications

Jackson, S. & Sachdev, D. (2001) *Better Education, Better Futures: Research, Practice and the Views of Young People in Public Care*, Barnardo's, Ilford.

Martín, E., Muñoz, C., Rodríguez, T. & Pérez, Y. (2008) 'De la residencia a la escuela: la integración social de los menores en acogimiento residencial con el grupo de iguales en el contexto escolar', *Psicothema*, vol. 20, no. 3, pp. 376–382.

Montserrat, C. (2008) *Niños, niñas y adolescentes acogidos por sus familiares: ¿qué sabemos, qué conocemos? [Children in kinship care. What do we know?]*, Generalitat de Catalunya, Barcelona.

Montserrat, C. & Casas, F. (2007) 'Kinship foster care from the perspective of quality of life: research on the satisfaction of the stakeholders', *Applied Research in Quality of Life*, vol. 1, pp. 227–237.

Montserrat, C. & Casas, F. (2010) 'Educación y jóvenes ex-tutelados: revisión de la literatura científica española', *Educación XX1*, vol. 13, no. 2, pp. 117–138.

Montserrat, C., Casas, F. & Bertran, I. (2010) *La situació escolar dels adolescents acollits en centre residencial, família extensa o aliena a Catalunya [The education of children in residential, kinship and foster care]*, [Online] Available at: http://www.udg.edu/eridiqv

Montserrat, C., González, M. & Malo, S. (2010) 'Podem identificar alguns factors d'èxit en l'acolliment d'infants i adolescents en els CRAE? [Can we identify some successful factors among children with a care background?]* Inf@ncia', *Butlletí dels professionals de la infància i l'adolescència*, vol. 41, pp. 1–6.

O'Sullivan, A. & Westerman, R. (2007) 'Closing the gap. Investigating the barriers to educational achievement for looked after children', *Adoption and Fostering*, vol. 31, no. 1, pp. 13–20.

Rutter, M. (2000) 'Children in substitute care: some conceptual considerations and research implications', *Children and Youth Services Review*, vol. 22, no. 9/10, pp. 685–703.

Secretaria de Joventut (Youth Secretariat). (2008) *Vulnerabilitat dels joves davant la crisi [Vulnerable young people and the cirsis]*, Generalitat de Catalunya, Barcelona.

Shlonsky, A. & Berrick, J. (2001) 'Assessing and promoting quality in kin and nonkin foster care', *Social Service Review*, vol. 3, pp. 6–83.

Sinclair, I., Baker, C., Lee, J. & Gibbs, I. (2007) *The Pursuit of Permanency. A Study of the English Child Care System*, Jessica Kingsley, London.

Stein, M. & Munro, E. (eds.) (2008) *Young People's Transitions from Care to Adulthood, International Research and Practice*, Jessica Kingsley Publishers, London.

Tajfel, H. (1984) *Grupos humanos y categorías sociales [Human groups and social categories]*, Herder, Barcelona.

Ward, H., Munro, E. & Dearden, C. (2006) *Babies and Young Children in Care: Life Pathways, Decision-Making and Practice*, Jessica Kingsley Publishers, London.

Ward, H., Skuse, T. & Munro, E. R. (2005) '"The best of times, the worst of times". Young people views of care and accommodation', *Adoption and Fostering*, vol. 29, no. 1, pp. 8–17.

School as an opportunity and resilience factor for young people placed in care

Skolans betydelse för livschanser och motståndskraft hos barn och unga placerade i familjehem eller HVB-hem

Ingrid Höjer & Helena Johansson

The aim of this article is to describe and discuss how school can constitute a life opportunity and a resilience factor for young people at risk, as well as for those placed in care. Thirty-three young people were interviewed on two separate occasions. The results showed that school could provide a place of structure and safety, in contrast to a chaotic family life. When it was impossible to bring friends home, due to parents' problems, school also gave young people from dysfunctional families a chance to spend time with friends, and provided them with a sense of 'normality'. When school had skilled professionals—teachers, mentors and nurses—who approached children and young people with empathy and commitment, our interviewees felt recognised and appreciated. The possibility of repeating a year was also of importance. Providing a school of high as well as stable quality, with well educated and committed professionals, may constitute an important resilience factor for disadvantaged children and young people, and thus constitute a platform for the opening of educational pathways and enhancing of future life opportunities. School could also give children and young people access to social capital, when birth families had few resources.

Syftet med denna artikel är att beskriva och diskutera de sätt på vilka utbildning kan utgöra en livsmöjlighet och en resilient faktor för unga i riskzonen, likaväl som för de som placerats i samhällsvård. 33 ungdomar intervjuades vid två skilda tillfällen (26 deltog vid andra tillfället). Resultaten visar att skolan kan utgöra en strukturerad och trygg plats, i kontrast till en kaotisk familjesituation. När det, beroende på föräldrarnas problem, var omöjligt att ta hem kamrater kunde skolan ge ungdomarna från dysfunktionella familjer möjligheten att umgås med vänner och utveckla en känsla av 'normalitet'. I skolor, med utbildade professionella—lärare, mentorer, skolsköterskor— som mötte barnen och ungdomarna med empati och engagemang, kände sig intervjupersonerna sedda och uppskattade. Möjligheten att gå om ett år var också viktigt för dem. Tillgång till utbildning av hög och jämn kvalitet, med välutbildade och engagerade professionella, kan utgöra en viktig resilient faktor för utsatta barn och ungdomar och därmed skapa en plattform för högre utbildning och stärkta framtida livsmöjligheter. Skolan kunde också ge tillgång till socialt kapital när ursprungsfamiljerna saknade sådana resurser.

Introduction

Good school results are more than ever stressed as the key to a good life. Due to an increased level of education among the general population, young people with low educational attainments are at risk of facing severe problems in the labour market.

A report from the Swedish Board of Health and Welfare (National Board of Health and Welfare, 2010) shows that marks from the final year in compulsory school (9th form) have decisive significance for children's readiness to later continue on to higher education. About 20–30% of children with low marks or incomplete compulsory education leave school before having completed secondary education, compared to <1% of children with marks above the average. This concerns especially so-called disadvantaged children and among them are children raised in public care. They are, as a group, known to leave compulsory school with far lower marks than other children (Dixon *et al.*, 2004; Vinnerljung *et al.*, 2005; Cameron, 2007; Courtney *et al.*, 2007; National Board of Health and Welfare, 2010). Low marks may prevent them from being accepted on any of the national programmes at upper secondary school. Furthermore, research shows that children who grow up in care often leave upper secondary school with significantly lower marks than other children, or drop out of upper secondary school without any certificates. Of individuals born between 1972 and 1992 in Sweden, 60% of those who were placed in care, or had previous experiences of being in care, dropped out of secondary school, whereas for peers without care experience the corresponding figure was 18% (Johansson *et al.*, 2011).

Register studies carried out at the National Board of Health and Welfare, have aroused an increased awareness in Sweden of the importance of supporting children and young people placed in public care to perform well at school. If future prospects for children in care are to be improved, it is vital to find out what factors at school are perceived as positive and supportive by the children and young people themselves. In the recently completed research study *Young People from a Public Care Background: Pathways to Education in Europe* (YIPPEE), the overall aim was to investigate the educational pathways of young men and women from a public care background in five EU countries.[1] In this article, drawing mainly on findings from the Swedish part of the study, we aim to describe and discuss how school can constitute a life opportunity and a resilience factor for young people *at risk,* as well as for those placed in care. Why we chose to include both young people *at risk* and *placed in care,* may need a more thorough explanation. In the YIPPEE project, all our interviewees had experience of placements in care, and the aim of the project was, as mentioned earlier, to explore educational pathways of young people who had been in public care as children. However, it is important to remember that most of these young people experienced a problematic life before they were taken into care (23 out of 33 were placed in care after their 10th birthday). In the interviews our informants told us of dysfunctional family life—mainly due to parents' (most frequently single mothers) mental illness and/or drug and alcohol abuse. Frequent moves with their families meant equally frequent changes of schools—and thus disrupted relations with teachers, classmates and friends. Therefore we cannot limit our aim to comprise only experiences while *in care,* we also need to include the experiences of our informants before they entered care, although in this article the main focus is on the time when the children and young people were looked after away from home.

The Swedish Context

Education

In Sweden, it is compulsory to spend nine years at school—from 7 to 16 years of age. Upper secondary school is free, non-compulsory schooling for young people aged 16–19, and consists of 17 national programmes. The upper secondary school comprises three years and is not compulsory by law, but in practice is considered to be obligatory.

Nine in ten of all students who leave compulsory school are qualified to enter upper secondary school (Swedish National Agency for Education, 2011). For those who are not qualified, there are special programmes where they can work to improve their grades, or follow specially designed curricula for their time in upper secondary school. As a consequence, almost all young people are considered to be included in the upper secondary school system.

All those with the right educational qualifications are encouraged to continue their studies at university level or equivalent. There are no tuition fees, and study loans from the state (without security) to cover the cost of living are easily accessible. In 2008, the loan sum was approximately 187 Euros a week (40 weeks a year) of which 123 Euros are to be paid back.

Public Care

About 23,400 Swedish children and young people were placed in care at some time during 2009 (National Board of Health and Welfare, 2010). Of these, 17,900 were placed voluntarily under the Social Services Act, 6100 were placed on a mandatory care order under the Care of Young People Act, and 2200 were placed in emergency care. For those placed on a mandatory care order, 50% were in care due to care deficits in the home, 40% were in care due to their own behaviour (dysfunctional, antisocial and criminal behaviour) and 10% were in care due to a combination of these reasons. About 70% of the 23,400 in care are over 13 years old, which may be explained by the fact that youth justice is included in the child welfare system in Sweden. As the majority are placed in care after their 13th birthday, many young people are likely to have experienced difficulties and traumatic events prior to the placement. Over recent decades, about 75% of all children and young people in care have been placed in foster families. Foster care has been the preferred option as opposed to residential care; the familial context is believed to give a child or young person the most favourable environment.

A young person in Sweden normally leaves care when he/she reaches the age of 18 or when he/she finishes upper secondary school—this is usually at the age of 19. After leaving care, the extended responsibility from society ceases. At that point the young person is considered 'like anyone else' and has to apply for support (economic, practical, etc.) through the same channels and with the same form of assessment as other adults, independently of background. Most local authorities embrace a policy whereby young people can stay in care, without interruption, until they have finished upper secondary school even if they are 19 or more—but this is not mandatory, and some authorities have been known to end the placement at the point when the young person reaches 18 years old (Höjer & Sjöblom, 2010), regardless of the stage they have reached in their education.

Previous Knowledge

Educational achievements of children and young people placed in care have, until recently, received little or no attention in Sweden. Vinnerljung (1998) calls attention to the absence of Swedish research directed towards foster children and their educational attainments. He comments that this lack of interest is hard to explain, as child welfare legislation in Sweden for decades has been highlighting the importance of foster children's educational attainments (Vinnerljung, 1998).

Results from Swedish research show that young people formerly placed in care are less likely to perform well at school, and their chances of moving on to further and higher education are limited, compared to their peers (Vinnerljung *et al.*, 2005). In cohorts 1972–1992, 14% of children and young people placed in care did not finish compulsory school at all, compared to 3% of their peers with no experience of a placement in care (Johansson *et al.*, 2011). Furthermore, of those who left compulsory school in 2007, 4% of the majority population did not have a pass in

Swedish, 6% did not have a pass in English and the corresponding figure for Mathematics was 7%. For those who had been placed in care, 18% did not have a pass in Swedish, 24% did not have a pass in English, and as many as 28% did not have a pass in Mathematics. Furthermore, for cohorts 1972–1992, 13% of those with experience of placements in care were registered at university, compared to 41% of the majority population (Johansson *et al.*, 2011). Even though less successful school performance may be explained by difficulties connected to children's and young people's situation *pre care*, it is still a fact that a placement in care has not compensated young people for previous difficulties and shortcomings at school (Jackson & Sachdev, 2001; Social Exclusion Unit, 2003; Vinnerljung *et al.*, 2005; Pecora *et al.*, 2006).

A substantial amount of research on children and young people in care and their school performance is focused on problems and shortcomings related to school (Vinnerljung, 1998; Jackson & Sachdev, 2001; Vinnerljung *et al.*, 2005; National Board of Health and Welfare, 2010;). However, there are also research findings reporting on support in relation to educational achievements. For example, Harker *et al.* (2003) found teachers to be frequent providers of support for children and young people placed in care. In this study children in residential care seemed to have more access to educational support, compared to those placed in foster care (Harker *et al.*, 2003) Happer *et al.* (2006) identifies some factors which had an impact on looked after young people's success at school: high expectations from teachers as well as from carers, stability of placement and being seen as someone who could achieve.

Social problems continuing from adolescence into adulthood are often connected to personal resources. If the accumulation of problems in the child's life could be reduced, this also reduces the risk of problems occurring later in life (Stattin & Magnusson, 1996). Gilligan (2000) argues for the use of the concept of *resilience* as an organising concept in work with children in need (Gilligan, 2000, p. 37). The concept of resilience is defined by Rutter (1999) as a capacity to overcome difficult life experiences. According to Stein (2005), recent empirical research has focused on three main areas of resilience: the attributes of children and young people themselves; their family relationships; and the characteristics of their wider social environments. For young people from very disadvantaged family backgrounds, the capacity of resilience was connected to having a trusting relationship with a member of family or other significant person, a feeling of being in control of their lives, positive school experiences and being given the opportunity of a 'turning point' to change a negative life course (Rutter *et al.*, 1998). This is in concordance with Gilligan (2000; 2007), who found that good school achievements, good and trusting relations to teachers, as well as access to spare time activities, greatly improved the self-esteem and -efficacy of young people in care who had previously experienced adversity.

However, although the perspective of resilience is of great importance, it is also vital not to over-emphasise the capacity for resiliency. Both Ungar (2001) and Samuels and Pryce (2008) describe how young persons in public care construct their identities in relation to two discourses; vulnerable and needy on the one hand and on the other resilient and independent. A strong resilient identity can also have a negative aspect, leading young people not to ask for or receive support from a social network or other supporting structures such as the social services even when they really need it. Social workers and other professionals have an important role in enhancing a feasible identity position of the young persons. This means navigating between acknowledging vulnerability, dependency and extraordinary experiences and, at the same time, supporting a strong sense of autonomy and resilience.

The concept of *social capital* can give us an understanding of how access to different kinds of support can have an impact on young people's lives. The amount of social capital which a person has acquired, i.e. people or groups who can be relied upon in specific situations, has an important influence on the creation, or strengthening, of an individual's resilience. *Social capital* can be categorised as *bonding* and *bridging*. Bonding social capital refers to the relationships and networks that consist of trust and reciprocity and that reinforce bonds in the social network. The cornerstone here is to strengthen the ties within the network. Bridging social capital emphasises the importance of connections that link networks across different heterogeneous groups (Helve & Bynner, 2007). Support not only from parents, but also from schools and communities, are expressions of useful social capital (Pinkerton & Dolan, 2007). Positive forms of bonding social capital can provide a stable identity and help young people to bridge out of disadvantaged family situations to connect with more heterogeneous groups (Holland, 2007).

Method

In studying pathways to post-compulsory education several different methods were used; secondary data, literature review, interviews with managers of social services, and interviews with young people in care and additionally adults nominated by them as having been supportive to their educational progress. In the analysis of secondary data, two datasets were combined for the first time; GOLD from the Department of Education, University of Gothenburg and data from the National Board of Health and Welfare concerning measures taken/interventions for children and youth.[2]

The sample of young people participating in the interview study was drawn from different local authority areas of West Sweden. To be eligible for the study, the young people were supposed to fit the following criteria: being 18–21 years of age, having spent at least one year in care, being in care at the age of 16, and showing educational promise. The criterion of 'educational promise' was hard to apply similarly in the five participating countries, due to different school systems. In Sweden, we decided that 'educational promise' could be defined as having a pass in Swedish, English and Mathematics at compulsory school. A pupil with a pass in these three subjects would be eligible for acceptance at upper secondary school.

A total of 333 letters were sent out to young people in the selected local authorities. About 53 screening interviews were performed at a first stage, and eventually 33 young people who fitted the criteria agreed to do a face-to-face interview. Although the sample, according to these procedures, may be considered as self selected, it constitutes an important source of information on the young people's personal experiences. However, these 33 young people cannot be regarded as representative of the whole population: firstly, because they were selected as 'educationally promising', secondly they had to take an active step in order to become part of the interviewed group. As an example of the difference between the 33 young people in the sample, and the total population found when joining the two data-sets, it can be mentioned that 24 out of 33 (72%) were young women compared to 49% in the national statistical data. Furthermore, 7 (21%) were in higher education at the time of the interview while this was the case for only 14% in the joint data. Later, 26 follow-up telephone interviews were conducted, as well as interviews with nominated adults. All interviews were recorded, transcribed and analysed using the NVIVO software program.

Methodological Considerations

The criterion of *educational promise* intentionally produced a sample which is not representative of all children placed in care but only of those who appear to have the potential to progress to higher levels of education. We wanted to find out if they did in fact do so and if not what were the obstacles that stood in their way. Figures from register studies presented earlier, clearly show that a high proportion of young people who have been placed in care, or still are in care, do not fit the criteria for the Swedish sample. Consequently, we can expect the young people in our sample to have a more positive attitude towards school, and also towards teachers and the learning process as a whole.

The low response rate for the letters sent out to the young people—approximately 14%—also implies that the sample cannot be considered as representative. Furthermore, our impression is that some young people were willing to participate in the study because they had been approached by social workers, foster carers or residential staff, with whom they had a good relationship. Therefore, it is possible that our sample may only consist of young people with positive experiences of the care system, and we might have failed to reach those with more negative experiences.

Additionally, in Sweden many enter into higher education late in life seen from a European perspective. This suggests that a group of young persons who do not fit the YIPPEE criteria (because they do not achieve the required standard at the end of compulsory schooling) may still, in the future, be found at our universities. This, by definition, is a group that we have failed to reach and it would have required a much longer follow-up period to do so.

Results

School As Haven—And a Chance To Be 'Like Everyone Else'

Many of our respondents shared similar experiences of family life before they were taken into care. A summarised, and somewhat generalised, description of the family situation for a high proportion of our respondents would be as follows: single mother with low level of education, often unemployed or on sick leave, weak networks, violence in the home, alcohol and/or drug abuse, together with mental illness. This meant that family life was often chaotic, without any structure. Such an environment provided little support for school attainments. Furthermore, many of the interviewed young people had to take responsibility for their younger siblings as well as for their parents. This left little time for home-work, and also hindered them from seeing friends.

As a contrast to such a disorganised setting at home, for many of our respondents school represented structure, calm and a chance to meet adults who supported them in different ways. School also meant a hot and nourishing meal every day—school lunches were an important complement when there was no food at home. One of our informants, Edith, who was homeless for three years—staying with different friends—described school as her secure base, where she felt safe and recognised. For her, school was a haven, where she met adults who took an interest in her.

Anna grew up with her mother, and four younger siblings. The mother lived in several destructive relationships, which included severe mental and physical abuse. Anna's mother had problems in providing a secure financial situation for herself and her children. Like Edith, Anna described school as her secure place even though she was bullied. For Anna, school was a contrast to the chaotic situation she experienced at home:

> School has always been a good thing, it was only in 8th grade that I started skipping classes because I couldn't take more. But when I did go, I didn't want to go home from school.

Several of the young people also told us how they perceived themselves as 'different' from their peers. Due to the problematic situation at home, they could never bring friends to visit. Additionally, they felt they were dressed differently, and could not afford to take part in the same leisure activities as their friends did. In such cases, school could provide a sense of 'normality'. Indra described how her situation was normalised by competent school staff. She was a pupil among others, and could meet friends in a 'normal' setting. At school she did not have to feel ashamed or embarrassed for her background or the fact that she now lived in a foster family. For Indra, school also created a much appreciated 'zone of normality'. Pekka came from a socially dysfunctional family, where he had experienced abuse and neglect. This caused him to feel embarrassed and different in relation to friends. In the interview, he often referred to how he appreciated school as a provider of 'normality':

> I could be with normal people, attend a normal school, have normal classes and see normal friends.

Indra and Pekka are good examples of how school may serve as an arena where differences and inequalities could be limited. Positive social capital, not accessible in the birth family, or in the foster family, could be accessible at school. However, such positive experiences also depend on a safe environment at school, and supportive and empathetic professionals.

Having a Second Chance

Several of our informants told us of long periods of absence from school, usually before they came into care. Such periods could be due to depression, bullying, or sometimes be related to problems in the family. On such occasions, the *possibility of getting back on track* was crucial. For our informants, the importance of this possibility cannot be overestimated. Without it many of them would probably not have continued their educational career. Pekka, constitutes a good example of the significance of such a second chance. He was taken into care due to severe physical abuse by his birth mother, and placed in a foster family where both foster parents were teachers. When taken out of the special education group, where he had been placed because of his behavioural problems, he repeated his fourth year in a 'normal' class. With support from his new foster family, Pekka could start all over and eventually had no problems at school. He even became chairman of the pupils' board and a peer helper. He continued his commitment at upper secondary school and finished with good grades. He now plans to become a policeman or a social worker but wants to work for a couple of years before starting his higher education. Having the opportunity to leave special education and repeat a year in an ordinary class has meant a lot to him:

> I could repeat one year, because I was a little bit behind. So when I was eleven I started fourth grade. And since then it's worked really well. The whole schooling has been ... I caught up everything in, I don't know, maybe half a year, I caught up with everything, I was among the best at maths and a lot of things.

Being Competent

In the interviews many young persons described compulsory school as a positive experience, which often implied a *feeling of being able, being smart*, and as someone to whom *'everything comes easy'*. Some describe how specific subjects really appealed to them, which made them achieve well, and thus also feel clever and capable. Surprisingly many of the young persons interviewed described themselves as good at school, smart, talented or in other positive terms. Their educational identity was strong and positive. During the interviews a number of positive stories were told of experiences which reinforced their sense of themselves as being capable and learning persons.

Such a strong learning identity was an important part of their self-image, and like Eva in the following quotation, our informants were aware of their competence, which was described as an inner capacity, a personal incentive to perform, without the support from parents they perceived as available for their peers:

> I've always liked school, thought it was fun and . . . I don't know if it was in second grade but the teacher suggested that I should skip a grade because I was so far ahead of all the rest . . . I was a quick learner . . .

Additionally, teachers' expressed perception of them as gifted and intelligent helped create a positive self-image and a positive attitude towards school. The majority of the young persons expressed such a positive attitude, at least during part of their compulsory schooling. This feeling must be characterised as one factor supporting school attendance and motivation.

Siri experienced placement breakdown in her early teens. Her school attainments were poor, and she had a record of truancy. Eventually she was placed with committed carers, who put a strong emphasis on school attendance achievement. She shared the experience of being seen and encouraged:

> I had the best attendance. And like, we were four girls who went to France, we were the best four that went as trainees for a month. So I felt that I was successful all the time, because I got something for it.

Siri described how she was seen by her teachers in a positive and affirmative way. (This was not at all the case in her previous school). In interaction with people around her she got to hear, and experience, that she was a good learner and integrated that description of herself as part of her identity. She managed to take a position where she constructed herself as successful, valued and capable. This position, when taken, tends to reward itself and thus becomes strengthened.

Being Seen

Another positive factor detected in the empirical material is a sense of *being seen*. Several young persons described a mentor, an assistant, a teacher or someone else within school who recognised them and saw them as individuals. We have examples from the interviews where the young people tell us of teachers extending their pedagogic task to also include a commitment to the social situation of the young person. Camilla emphasised the importance of such a person being familiar with her home situation:

> I had Esther, my mentor. We had her from sixth to ninth grade and she came to a lot of meetings with the social services and everything. She knew everything about mum and things, so she was always . . . She helped me with maths when I needed, and so on. She was always there. So a lot of things are thanks to her, too.

Anders received great support from the school nurse during a very turbulent time in his life:

> I was never at school, she was the only one that noticed. [. . .]When I needed to talk, I went to see her. And she always found time and talked to me and . . . Like, even if she had a break she talked to me.

Several other interviewees tell similar stories of adults at school, not necessarily teachers, but also for example school meals staff and recreation centre assistants, who made the young persons feel seen, respected and listened to. Such recognition from school staff could make the difference between school as a negative and positive experience.

School As Platform For A Better Life

Many of the young women and men, express their dreams and goals in very powerful ways. They have dreams and aspirations, they plan for the future, and show a lot of drive in relation to continued studies. Eva, who is at university doing social work, answers the question 'Have you always known what you wanted to do?':

> I've always had it set out for me, kind of. Like, now I'll do this and then that. So, there hasn't been any question about it.

Jessica, who has fought hard to enter into nursing at university, paints two pictures, two alternatives she can envisage for herself; one picture represents a monotonous job in a grocery store, unpacking goods, the other a stimulating lifelong job:

> And what do you get then, you get full time at a shitty place, at Lidl or something. It gives money but it doesn't give any satisfaction working, it's like slavery, you go like a robot. I think it's extremely important that you work in something you like. You'll work there, like, most part of your life.

Another distinct theme in the interviews is a strong and manifest determination not to end up where their parents or relatives are. The determination and force to *break with a social legacy* are strong and can be expressed in terms of resistance, dissociation or revenge. Anna develops her thoughts on where her will to succeed comes from:

> I guess it's my own determination, I mean, hello, I don't want to become, I've got an aunt who's a junkie and alcoholic, I don't want to be like her, I've got an uncle who's an ex junkie, a granny who's an alcoholic and two other uncles who're criminals and batterers and God knows what. I don't want to become like them.

Several young persons participating in the study told us of how they have managed to turn severe problems at home during childhood into a certain sense of strength, which they can benefit from for the rest of their lives. They have made it against all odds. At least for some of the young people interviewed, school seems to have succeeded in becoming a place where they have felt encouraged and normal, despite their background, and where some important cornerstones for further education have been laid. Thus, school has created a platform from which these young people can start to build a better life for themselves.

Supporting Adults—Access to Social Capital

Each one of the 33 young persons interviewed was asked to nominate one adult person who had supported them in their educational life. About 25 of these 33 were able to nominate one such person. They were 13 foster carers, six teachers, three birth mothers, two residential staff and one counsellor. Support in educational matters may be connected to access to social capital. The nominated adults in our sample provided our interviewees with information and knowledge about the educational system. Having the opportunity to discuss educational pathways was of great importance for the young people, as was support and encouragement of school achievements. Very few (three) of our informants had access to such social capital and support from their birth families. Thus, the 'nominated adults' provided them with an important source of social capital. Seven young persons had no access to social capital in this form and could not think of anyone who had acted as provider of support or given them encouragement.

However, a substantial proportion (12 out of 15) of the young persons interviewed who had taken a 'straight' educational pathway through secondary education could identify one or more persons who had provided them with support in school achievements. Three (out of the 15) could not and Julia states, with emphasis 'I have tried to manage on my own and without any support'.

Discussion

This study focuses on a vulnerable and exposed group of children who, as young adults, tell their stories of poverty, negligence, abuse, maltreatment and insecurity. They carry all signs of being at risk of having serious problems as adults. By choosing to interview a number of young persons that, in spite of their background, have 'made it' and are showing educational promise, the study has set out to investigate factors and circumstances that support this positive development.

One of the factors important for the capacity of being resilient is a feeling of being in control (Rutter *et al.*, 1998). School as a provider of structure meant that our informants had a sense of being in control of their lives, in contrast to the powerlessness they could experience in their birth families, as well as in care placements. When school staff could offer empathy and support, this helped the young people to sort out their accomplishments at school. One might say that such support helped our informants to 'interpret' school as a system, understand what was needed to perform well, and bask in the praise which followed good achievements. They were in control, they could make plans and feel capable, which enhanced their capacity to be resilient.

As described previously, many of our young informants perceived themselves as being 'different'. At school, the feeling of being different was not as manifest, and they could feel 'normal', as one in the peer group. The time they spent at school could perhaps be described as some kind of 'intermission' in an often chaotic life, where the stigmatic burden of coming from a dysfunctional family or being placed in care could be taken off their shoulders. Apparently, this had a tangible effect on their sense of well-being and also on their capacity to achieve at school. Thus, it enhanced their resiliency.

The concept of social capital is also applicable to the situation of our informants. The access to social capital, *bonding* as well as *bridging*, is important to create a stable identity (Helve & Bynner, 2007; Pinkerton & Dolan, 2007). In many cases, the young people we have interviewed had little access to positive social capital. Relations to family members, and sometimes also to carers, could be complicated or negative. Additionally, access to sustaining networks was seldom available. When our informants described support from professionals at school, such support provided them with a kind of social capital, not supplied by family or carers. In those cases, school compensated for the lack of social capital, and thus enhanced a positive identity and self-perception for the young people.

Conclusion

Children and young people spend a great deal of their childhood and adolescence at school, and their interaction with professionals and peers is likely to have a tangible impact on self esteem and identity. In the interviews, our respondents did not always describe school as idyllic. Several informants mentioned bullying, both by teachers and peers, and feelings of exclusion. However, in this article we have aimed at describing how school can provide an opportunity and act as a factor in promoting resilience. We have tried to show how school can be a positive and empowering experience for young people from different types of disadvantaged backgrounds. Although in this article we have focused on those in care, or who later came into care, it applies equally to those not in care who come from similarly troubled families.

When schools had skilled professionals—teachers, mentors and nurses—who approached children and young people with empathy and commitment, our interviewees felt recognised and appreciated. A majority of those who managed to move on to college or university told us about being seen and supported by school professionals. Furthermore, when school provided a safe and secure environment, our interviewees could use school as a haven, as compensation for a lack of security and attention at home. The possibility of repeating a year when their school attendance had been disrupted by family upheavals or by coming into care had also been of great importance to some of our informants.

In conclusion, it is possible to argue that if society's aim of preventing social exclusion of vulnerable and exposed children and young people is to be successful, school should be a key area for intervention. Providing a stable placement in a school of high quality, with well educated and committed professionals, may constitute an important resilience factor for disadvantaged children and young people, especially those in public care, and thus be a platform for the opening of educational pathways and, by its extension, enhancing their future life opportunities.

Notes

[1]   The research leading to these results received funding from the European Union's Seventh Framework Programme under Grant agreement no. 217297. The research project was undertaken by a team of cross-national researchers from: the Danish School of Education University of Aarhus, Denmark; the Institute for Social Policy and Labour, Hungary; the Research Institute on Quality of Life, University of Gerona, Spain; the Department of Social Work and the Department of Education, University of Gothenburg; and the Thomas Coram Research Unit, Institute of Education, University of London, England. All the researchers have contributed to the research reported here but responsibility for this article lies with the authors. The views expressed in this article are those of the authors and not necessarily those of other partners or of the European Union.

[2]   GOLD includes all individuals born between 1972 and 1992, who lived in Sweden at the age of 16. ($N = 2,184,866$). The data-set contains for example data on parents' education, family structure and information of the educational situation of the individual (all forms of schools, grades, programmes at university, exams, study financing etc.). There are some limitations; data after the completion of compulsory school are missing for the cohorts born 1988–1992. Statistics on measures taken/interventions by the social services for children and young persons have since 1994 been published by the National Board of Health and Welfare. The statistics contain data on all young persons placed in care, including legal framework, time in care, age at first placement, number of placements and placement form (foster home or residential care). In the sample used within the project persons born 1973 and later were included.

References

Cameron, C. (2007) 'Education and self-reliance among care leavers', *Adoption and Fostering*, vol. 3, no. 1, pp. 39–49.

Courtney, M., Dworsky, A., Gretchen, R., Havlicek, J., Perez, A. & Keller, T. (2007) *Midwest Evaluation of the Adult Functioning of Former Foster Youth: Outcomes at age 21*, Chapin Hall Center for Children, The University of Chicago, Chicago.

Dixon, J., Wade, J. & Weatherley, H. (2004) *Young People Leaving Care: A Study of Outcomes and Costs*, Social Work Research and Development Unit, University of York, York.

Gilligan, R. (2000) 'Adversity, resilience and young people: The protective value of positive school and spare time experiences', *Children and Society*, vol. 14, pp. 37–47.

Gilligan, R. (2007) 'Adversity, resilience and the educational progress of young people in public care', *Emotional and Behavioural Difficulties*, vol. 12, no. 2, pp. 135–145.

Happer, H., Mc Creaide, J. & Aldgate, J. (2006) *Celebrating Success: What Helps Looked After Children Succeed*, Social Work Inspection Agency, Edinburgh, UK.

Harker, R., Dobel-Ober, D., Lawrence, J., Berridge, D. & Sinclair, R. (2003) 'Who takes care of education? Looked after children's perceptions of support for educational progress', *Child and Family Social Work*, vol. 8, no. 1, pp. 89–100.

Helve, H. & Bynner, J. (2007) 'Youth and social capital', in *Youth and Social Capital*, eds H. Helve & J. Bynner, The Tufnell Press, London, pp. 1–11.

Höjer, I. & Sjöblom, Y. (2010) 'Young people leaving care in Sweden', *Child and Family Social Work*, vol. 15, pp. 118–127.

Holland, J. (2007) 'Inventing adulthoods: Making the most of what you have', in *Youth and Social Capital*, eds H. Helve & J. Bynner, The Tufnell Press, London, pp. 11–28.

Jackson, S. & Sachdev, D. (2001) *Better Education, Better Futures: Research, Practice and the Views of Young People in Public Care*, Barnardo's, Ilford.

Johansson, H., Höjer, I. & Hill, M. (2011) 'Young people from a public care background and their pathways to education – final report from the Swedish part of the YIPPEE project', Available at http://www.socwork.gu.se/forskning/forskningsprogram_famlij/Yippee/

National Board of Health and Welfare. (2010) *Social Rapport 2010*, National Board of Health and Welfare, Stockholm.

Pecora, P., Kessler, R., O'brien, K., Roller White, C., Williams, J., Hirpi, E., English, D., White, J. & Herrick, M. A. (2006) 'Educational and employment outcomes of adults formerly placed in foster care: Results from the Northwest Foster Care Alumni Sudy', *Children and Youth Services Review*, vol. 28, pp. 1459–1481.

Pinkerton, J. & Dolan, P. (2007) 'Family support, social capital, resilience and adolescent coping', *Child and Family Social Work*, vol. 12, pp. 219–228.

Rutter, M. (1999) 'Resilience concepts and findings: Implications for family therapy', *Journal of Family Therapy*, vol. 21, pp. 119–144.

Rutter, M., Giller, H. & Hagell, A. (1998) *Antisocial Behaviour by Young People*, Cambridge University Press, Cambridge.

Samuels, G. M. & Pryce, J. M. (2008) '"What doesn't kill you makes you stronger": Survivalist self-reliance as resilience and risk among young adults aging out of foster care', *Children and Youth Services Review*, vol. 30, pp. 1198–1210.

Social Exclusion Unit. (2003) *A Better Education for Children in Care*, SEU, London.

Stattin, H. & Magnusson, D. (1996) 'Antisocial development: A Holistic approach', *Development and Psychopathology*, vol. 8, pp. 617–645.

Stein, M. (2005) *Resilience and Young People Leaving Care: Overcoming the odds*, Joseph Rowntree Foundation, ORT.

Swedish National Agency for Education. (2011) '*Elever som ej uppnått målen i ämnen som krävs för grundläggande behörighet, läsåren 2005/06-2009/10* [Students Not Reaching Required Goals in Subjects Needed for General Acceptance]' [Online] Available at: http://www.skolverket.se/content/1/c6/02/24/14/Grundskolan_Betygochprov_Riksniv%E5Tabell5webb.xls

Ungar, M. (2001) 'The social construction of resilience among "problem" youth in out-of-home placement: A study of health-enhancing deviance', *Child and Youth Care Forum*, vol. 30, no. 3, pp. 137–154.

Vinnerljung, B. (1998) 'Fosterbarns skolgång [Schooling and education of foster children]', *Socialvetenskaplig tidskrift*, vol. 5, no. 1, pp. 58–80.

Vinnerljung, B., Öman, M. & Gunnarsson, T. (2005) 'Educational attainments of former child welfare clients – A Swedish national cohort study', *Journal of Social Welfare*, vol. 14, no. 4, pp. 265–276.

The importance of social relationships for young people from a public care background

Tidligere anbragte unge og betydningen af sociale relationer

Inge M. Bryderup & Marlene Q. Trentel

The purpose of this article is to show that social relationships and participation in communities are of central importance to promoting positive educational pathways for young people from a public care background. The article will explore what facilitates and hinders young people's educational pathways. In addition to a general description of facilitators and barriers, this article focuses primarily on the importance of social relationships. This is done with reference to an EU research project called Young people from a public care background: Pathways to education in Europe. *This article will show that young people's age at entry to care, pre-care experiences and in-care experiences influence their educational pathways. The article argues for the importance of professionals to be proactive in helping young people access and engage in social communities.*

I denne artikel belyses, hvilke faktorer der har en positiv indvirkning på unges uddannelsesforløb. Samtidig vil det blive undersøgt, hvilke faktorer der udgør en barriere i forhold til de unges uddannelsesforløb. Facilitatorer og barrierer vil blive diskuteret, og der vil være særligt fokus på sociale relationer, da der argumenteres for, at sociale relationer og deltagelse i sociale fællesskaber har afgørende betydning for tidligere anbragte unges uddannelsesforløb. Artiklen bygger på et multimetodisk EU forskning-

sprojekt 'Young people from a public care background pathways to education in Europe' (Tidligere anbragte unges uddannelsesforløb i Europa). Det konkluderes i artiklen, at de tidligere anbragte unges opvækst og anbringelsesforløb påvirker deres uddannelsesforløb. Det påpeges, at det er af afgørende betydning, at de professionelle støtter de unge i at skabe adgang til og deltage i sociale fællesskaber.

Introduction

Approximately 15,000 children and young people are placed in care in Denmark. The general tendency is that younger children are placed in foster families and older children are placed in residential care centres (Bryderup, 2005). Other placement opportunities include private residential care centres, own accommodation, 'ship project' and boarding schools. In 2009, 42% of all the children placed in care were aged 15- to 17-years-old followed by 24% who were 12- to 14-years-old. The remaining 34% of children in care were aged from birth to 11 years.

Generally there are several reasons for a placement of a child or young person. In 2009, the most cited reason for placing a child or young person in care was disharmony in the family as well as problem behaviour and/or adaptation problems among the children/young people (Ankestyrelsen, 2009). Reasons also include having grown-up in socially disadvantaged families with lack of resources, substance misuse and illness (Egelund et al., 2008; Petersen, 2010).

Previous research in Denmark has shown that young people in care or from a public care background are disadvantaged on a number of levels and they are also more likely than their peers to experience educational difficulties (Christoffersen, 1993; Mortensøn & Neerbek, 2008; Ottosen & Christensen, 2008). In EU countries for which data are available, young men and women from a public care background are over-represented in virtually every indicator of disadvantage including: poverty, housing, unemployment, criminal activity and teenage pregnancy (Petrie & Simon, 2006). Other studies have also found that pathways into formal education and employment for disadvantaged young people, particularly young people in and leaving care, are often significantly more limited in terms of access and opportunities for a range of reasons including lack of qualifications, dis-engagement and demotivation (Dixon, Wade, & Weatherley 2004; Jackson & Sachdev, 2001). There are few studies in Denmark that have focused upon the educational levels of young people from a public care background *after* compulsory school. These studies show that young people in care or from a public care background lag far behind the educational levels of their peers in the overall population. They tend not to finish compulsory school at the same speed as all young people and only a minority obtain qualifications beyond compulsory school (Andersen (red.), 2010; Melbye & Husted 2009). Our study confirms these findings as our results show that 16% of young people aged 18- to 22-years-old who have been in care at the age of 16 have not completed compulsory school compared to 6% of all young people the same age. In addition, our findings show that 40% of young people aged 27- to 30-years-old who have been in care at the age of 16 have completed a post-compulsory educational course compared with 80% of all young people at the same age. There have been no previous studies in Denmark that have explored barriers and facilitators for young people's educational pathways. Moreover no studies have combined quantitative and qualitative data in documenting the educational experience of young people with a background in public care.

This article is based on Danish findings from the EU research project YiPPEE, *Young people from a public care background: pathways to education in Europe.*[1] The project used a multi-method approach and in this article we draw on Danish findings from both quantitative and qualitative data in order to explore the barriers and facilitators that young people encounter.

We start by describing the approach and methods in the study. We then present some statistical data about young people from a public care background and their educational qualifications, comparing them with all young people. This is followed by a description of five ideal types that have been identified which serves as an analytic frame for the analysis. The facilitators and barriers the young people encounter will be discussed and this, in turn, will be followed by a discussion of why social relationships are so important. Finally, we will draw on sociological perspectives in a discussion of individualisation, social relationships and participation in social communities.

Approach and methods

In the Danish study, the data collection comprised a literature review, analyses of statistical data, five area case studies and face-to-face interviews with care managers in five local authorities. Seventy-five telephone screening interviews were carried out with young people, 35 in-depth interviews with young people aged 19–21 selected from the screening interviews,[2] 29 follow-up interviews with the same young people[3] and 14 interviews with nominated adults.[4] In this article, we will mainly draw on the results from the in-depth interviews with the young people.

The young people interviewed in this study were drawn from five local authority areas of Denmark. The criteria for selecting the young people in the local authorities included that they (1) were aged between 19- and 21-years-old at the time (end of 2008) and (2) were placed in care at their 16th birthday and had been in care for a minimum of 1 year. These criteria were adopted by all countries in the YiPPEE project.[5] The young people who agreed to participate in the study comprised 75 young people out of a possible 235.[6] A further selection procedure then took place based on young people showing 'educational promise'. The criteria for showing educational promise were having completed compulsory school and having started on or being just about to start on an educational course. These criteria were fulfilled by 60 young people. The YiPPEE project design required us to interview 35 young people in each country and these were chosen according to availability and geographical spread.

The in-depth sample consisted of 35 young people, 11 men and 24 women aged 20–23 years. Thirty-one described themselves as white, 3 as mixed race and 1 as Asian. Four young people were born outside Denmark but at the time of the interview they were all Danish citizens. Of the 35 young people, 51.5% had spent most of their placements in foster care, 31.4% in residential care centres and private residential care centres, 11.4% in residential care centres *and* foster care and 5.7% in other placements. The majority of the interviewed young people had entered the care system when they were between 12- and 14-years-old and the majority had spent more than 4 years in care.

In the Danish study (Bryderup & Trentel, 2010), a grounded theory inspired approach was used in analysing the interviews with the young people, meaning that the empirical data were treated very carefully and sensitively. Our analysis has been inspired by Glaser and Strauss' (1967) term 'ever-developing' (p. 32) which denotes the joint collection, coding and analysis of data for instance by using schemes of codes and concepts and by doing comparative analysis. As outlined by Glaser and Strauss, interviews should be read and reread several times. The research team continuously returned to read the transcribed interviews when discussing themes and findings. Reading through the interviews several times ensured that the themes derived from the study were grounded in the empirical data. By doing so we gained insight into patterns that would not have been possible to identify otherwise. This method of returning to the interviews on an ongoing basis also facilitated the identification of *five ideal types* of young people based on their educational pathways, which we shall return to later after having briefly outlined the educational attainment of young people from a public care background.

Facts about young people's educational level

The aim of this section is to show that young people from a public care background lag far behind the educational levels of their peers in the overall population. We will present some statistics based on our secondary analysis of statistics from Statistic Denmark (Bryderup, Trentel, & Kring, 2010). All statistics are based on data as of the 31 December 2006. Young people who were in care for the whole of their 16th year or more have been included. This criterion was chosen since it corresponds with the criterion for selecting young people for interviews. It means that the young people have been in care for a minimum of 1 year but it should be noted that they have usually spent a much longer time in care. Table 1 gives how the educational levels of young people from a public care background in Denmark compare to those in the general population.

The table demonstrates that young people from public care lag far behind the educational levels of their peers in the overall population. They do not finish

Table 1. The attainment levels of young people from a public care background in Denmark compared to young people from the general population.

	17- to 20-year-olds from a public care background (%)	17- to 20-year-olds from the general population (%)	27- to 30-year-olds from a public care background (%)	27- to 30-years-old from the general population (%)
Not completed compulsory school	17	3	12	1
Qualifications beyond compulsory school	3	18	40	80

compulsory school at the same time or to the same extent as young people from the general population and only a minority obtain qualifications beyond compulsory school compared to their overall age cohort. These findings are supported by national and international research (see, for example, Andersen (red.), 2010; Cameron, Jackson, Hauari, & Hollingworth, 2011; Casas, Montserrat, & Malo, 2010; Höjer et al., 2008; Höjer, Johansson, & Hill, 2010; Melbye & Husted, 2009; Rácz, Csák, & Korintus, 2010).

It might be suggested that care leavers are only delayed in obtaining qualifications. However, our analyses show it is actually the case that, even when further qualifications are eventually obtained, the rate is still very low compared to the general population.

These findings clearly demonstrate that young people from a public care background in Denmark face educational barriers. What barriers do the young people encounter? In what way do their schooling experiences, upbringing and placement history influence their educational pathways? In what way do social relationships play a role for the young people?[7]

In the following section we will discuss the five identified 'ideal types', based on analyses of differences in the young people's educational pathways. By comparing the ideal types we will discuss facilitators and barriers for the young people and show that social relationships are crucial for young people in order to promote positive educational pathways and for them to navigate in a modern world.[8]

Five ideal types

Having analysed all the interviews with young people, we have identified five ideal types of young people *based on differences in their educational pathways*. Inspired by Weber's concept of ideal types (1949), this is a device we have adopted as a means of analysing, interpreting and representing data. Weber defines an ideal type as formed by characteristics and elements of a given phenomenon but it is not meant to correspond to all of the characteristics of any one particular case. Weber wrote that an ideal type is formed by the one-sided accentuation of one or more points of view and by the synthesis of a great many diffuse, discrete, more or less present and occasionally absent concrete individual phenomena, which are arranged according to those one-sidedly emphasised viewpoints into a unified analytical construct (Weber, 1949, p. 90). An *ideal type* is an analytical construction that serves the investigator as a measuring rod to ascertain similarities as well as deviations in concrete cases. The concept of ideal types is hence used in our analysis as a tool and analytic frame constructed from the empirical data that are used to analyse the differences and similarities between the young people's educational pathways. Our analyses show that the ideal types are selective in relation to points of comparison and contrast between the young people in each ideal type. Each ideal type addresses a range of issues via patterns of similarity.

We have chosen to compare different parameters such as educational career, characteristics of the biological family and upbringing, placement history and daily life, relationships and leisure time in order to analyse the similarities and differences between the ideal types. There proved to be five ideal types constructed from the empirical data about educational pathways that will be given in Table 2 and described in detail afterwards. It should be noted that all young people were selected because they showed educational promise, however, two of the identified ideal types stand out, as the young people in these groups were more successful in fulfilling the educational promise that they had shown at age 16, and this is reflected in the names of the ideal types.

Table 2 presents the characteristics of the five ideal types identified in the Danish study.

By analysing and comparing these ideal types we find that there are a number of similarities and differences between them. The similarities and differences between the ideal types shed light on barriers and facilitators in general and further help to explain why some young people managed better than others. The table includes several characteristics of the identified ideal types that all play a part, however, in this article we do not attempt to explore them all in equal depth.[9] When comparing the ideal types we find that there are two groups of young people that stand out from the other groups because they have had a *'straight' and linear transition* from compulsory school to further education: those educational pathways leading towards (1) college or university and (2) vocational training and education. The main difference between the two groups lies in their choice of qualification. These two groups had some characteristics which stood out and which had influenced their educational pathways compared to the other groups.

Both these groups of young people had experienced a *stable time in compulsory school* with no bullying and/or changes of school. They also differ from the other three groups because although most of the young people in these groups, in common with the whole research sample, had divorced parents who misused alcohol, the parents of those in these groups were *better educated* than the parents of young people in the other groups. Furthermore, these parents were *more supportive* of their children's educational pathways. The study also revealed that the group of young people studying or aiming to study at college or university were more likely to have *a close relationship with their parents*. Their upbringing can be seen as less problematic

Table 2. Characteristics of the five ideal types.

The five ideal types	Educational career	Characteristic of biological family and upbringing	Placement career	Daily life, relationships, leisure time
Young people with 'promising' educational pathways in college or university 10 young people	Stable compulsory school Few have changed school No drop-outs No bullying Straight transition from compulsory school to further and higher education Now studying at college or university	Some divorced parents Alcohol misuse A few had looked after younger siblings	Most placed in foster care at an early age Some had experienced breakdown of placements No history of crime or drug abuse	Living in apartment Established social network Good and close relationship with biological parents Many friends Good relationship with foster family/carers All had leisure time interests
Young people with 'promising' educational pathways—vocational education and training six young people	Stable compulsory school Few had changed school No drop-outs No bullying Straight transition from compulsory school vocational education and training Employed/unemployed at the time	Divorced parents Alcohol misuse Few had looked after younger siblings Ill parents	Half placed in foster care and half placed in residential care—the majority at an old age Experienced breakdown of placements No history of crime or drug abuse	Living in apartment with partner Established social network Irregular contact with biological parents No contact with father Many friends Half of the young people speak of a good relationship with foster family/carers Few have leisure time interests
Young people with yo-yo pathways in education nine young people	Unstable compulsory school Change of school Drop-outs Bullying Working Unemployed	Divorced parents Violence Alcohol misuse Few had looked after younger siblings	Most placed in foster care at an old age Most had experienced placement breakdown Alcohol abuse	Living in apartment with partner Good contact with mother Little or no contact with father Little or no talk of friends Few have a good relationship with foster family/carers Few had leisure time interests

Table 2 (*Continued*)

The five ideal types	Educational career	Characteristic of biological family and upbringing	Placement career	Daily life, relationships, leisure time
Young people with 'delayed' educational pathways four young people	Unstable compulsory school Repeated a year in compulsory school No drop-outs in education Bullying Unemployed Studying vocational education and training	Divorced parents Violence Alcohol misuse Looking after younger siblings Mentally ill parents Ill parents	Most placed in foster care at an old age No breakdown Drug abuse	Living alone in apartment/or with partner Irregular contact to biological parents Little or no talk of friends Good relationship with foster family Few had leisure time interests
Young people with health problems dominating their educational pathways six young people	Unstable compulsory school Drop-outs Most were in education at the time	Divorced parents Violence Drug abuse Crime Incest	Temporary care Most placed in foster care at an old age Breakdown of placements Drug abuse Alcohol abuse	Still placed in care living in apartment Irregular contact with biological parents No contact with father Little or no talk of friends Little contact with professionals Few had leisure time interests

as compared with the other groups. Furthermore, most of the young people in this group had been placed in care at an early age and thus subject to *early intervention*. The research revealed that *a safe community with adults in whom the young people could confide and trust* was important in supporting their educational progress as well as other aspects of their development.

The two groups with more positive pathways all referred to friends and in particular those in college and university talked of close friends and of spending time with *friends in their leisure time*. These young people were also most likely to *have nominated an adult* who had supported them. It was also common for the young people belonging to the two groups with higher level pathways in education to reflect their nominated adult's educational level. The young people appeared to have been influenced as well as supported by their nominated adult. It was common for young people in both groups to have a social life and to engage in social communities. The following case will highlight some of the characteristics that are common for the young people belonging to the groups with 'promising' pathways.

Marie is one of the girls who was identified as belonging to the group of young people pursuing pathways towards college or university. She had a stable time in compulsory school and a straight transition to further education. She is now studying for a Bachelor in Pedagogy. She was placed in care at the age of six and stayed with the same foster family until she moved to her own apartment. She did not speak of any health problems, unlike many of the other young people. She had good contact with her biological parents who were both educated and whom she regarded as having been supportive. Her mother who holds a Masters in Coaching was nominated as a supportive adult. Marie talked a lot about spending time with friends and about one of her spare time pursuits—swimming.

Obstacles to educational progression

We have also identified some barriers to education based on the analysis of interviews with the young people. Such barriers were mainly found in the analysis of the interviews with young people in the groups of young people with: (1) 'yo-yo' pathways in education; (2) those with 'delayed' pathways in education and (3) those with health problems dominating their educational pathways.

The young people belonging to these three groups experienced an *unstable time in compulsory school*. They had often been *bullied* and had *changed schools* several times. The problems in school often started prior to placement in care. They had experienced long periods of non-attendance. They had also dropped out of various courses in further education and had not obtained any formal educational qualifications beyond compulsory school. These three groups had a *more problematic family background* than the other two groups. The young people's accounts reveal that their families were more disadvantaged. Violence, illness, drug abuse and incest featured in the young people's accounts of their family life. In most cases there was *no tradition of education* in the family and the young people were offered no educational support. Their *relationships with their parents were typically irregular* and some of the interviewed young people had no contact with their parents at all. According to the young people their parents did not have the capacity to be supportive.

These young people were mainly *placed in care at an older age* and had generally experienced many changes of placement. The research findings showed consistently that the young people in these three groups *lacked continuity in their lives.* It was common for them to have lived a relatively lonely life with no close relationships and with few, if any, people to support them. Furthermore, the instability which characterised their lives caused them to be socially as well as educationally disadvantaged. *Few talked of any friends* and likewise, *only a few spoke of contact with previous carers.* Moreover, they were much less likely than those in the first two groups to speak of *engaging in any leisure time activities.*

The following case highlights some of the characteristics that are common for these three groups: an unstable time in school, placement at an older age, unsupportive mother and lack of social relationships. Lilje belongs to the group of young people with health problems dominating their educational pathways. She showed a pattern of starting and dropping out of educational courses, also typical of the 'yo-yo' group.

Lilje attended five different compulsory schools and dropped out of seventh grade due to substance misuse. She noted that one school was aware of the situation in her home since a teacher brought her a packed lunch every day in fourth grade. Nevertheless, she was not placed in care until she was 13-years-old. She was introduced to substance misuse in her own home since her single mother, who was addicted to alcohol and pills, was of the opinion that Lilje should become accustomed to using alcohol and pills in the home instead of somewhere else. Lilje was only 12 when she tried amphetamines for the first time. She completed ninth grade and continued to business school. She dropped out of business school and started in 10th grade but then dropped out of 10th grade and started it again a little later but still did not complete it. She also started business school for a second time but again failed to complete the course. She moved in with a new boyfriend but it turned out to be a violent relationship and she ended it after 3½ years. She took up many unskilled jobs before starting vocational education and training. She did not speak of friends, family or previous carers and she seemed to live a rather isolated life without any leisure activities. Contact with her mother appeared to be irregular, and she was not able to nominate a supportive adult.

Our findings suggest that social relationships are one of the most important factors that influence the young people's pathways. Those young people who have good relationships with their families and friends and engage in leisure time activities and other social communities seem to be more likely to carry on studying and more likely to complete their studies.

Findings from the 35 in-depth interviews

Overall the findings of the study show that, typically, the interviewed young people from all groups were well aware that they had to lead their own life, take responsibility and make life decisions. They recognised that they needed to take responsible for their own lives, and that their pathways were not predetermined by past experiences. In other words, they had absorbed and taken on *individualised thinking*. That manifested itself through the young people's motivation for completing an education. When the young people were questioned about what they thought it would take to fulfil their ambitions they typically answered: 'It is down to myself and my own effort'. This research revealed two key interlinked explanations for choosing to study and gain qualifications beyond compulsory school: (1) not wanting to 'end up' like their parents and (2) getting well-paid and secure employment.

Across all five ideal types, many young people dissociate themselves from their parents. They explain that they had seen what kind of life their parents were living and linked it to the parents' low socio-economic status.[10] In general, the young people regarded *education as a tool to live a better life* and to 'get a good job'. The notion of becoming an educated person was dominant in the interviews. The young people were striving to be part of the norm and in this respect the norm meant holding a good job and contributing to society. In the young people's view, their parents did not adhere to such a norm since they rarely held a job. The desire to complete their education and become part of the norm was a driving force for the young people, they believed that their pathways were not predetermined by their parents' experiences. The following quote from one of the interviewed young women illustrates this point:

> I knew that I had to start an education [post-compulsory educational course], to get more disciplined and I knew that I wanted a future and not end up like my mother. I often thought that I wanted to be like others, I wanted to be normal, I did not want to be a nobody. (Maria)

The analysis shows that the young people were striving to become 'an educated person' and they were aware of the individual responsibility of leading their own life. The young people say that they know it is down to their will and motivation to achieve their goals. But at the same time the analysis showed that in order to discuss possibilities and to support all the choices they have to make, they need social relationships to sustain their lives. Overall the findings in this study show that many of the young people experienced an unstable time in school, grew up in families with major problems including alcohol and drug misuse, illness and disruptions. Their parents had no resources to care for their children. Relationships had often been inverted and the parents had come to expect and demand care and attention from their own children. There are many examples of young people in our study who had to look after younger siblings, do the shopping and the cooking. Many of the young people have experienced disruptions in families, change of school and change of placement. Many of the young people have had no long-term stable relationships with friends and family due to the many problems and changes that they have experienced. One young man told us that:

> The only people in my family who talk together are my grandma and my auntie. My mother does not talk with them. It is very limited. It is only when I visit my grandma or auntie. Otherwise we do not have any family (laughs). That was spoiled a long time ago. (Noah)

In this quote, Noah was referring to his mother's substance misuse that had resulted in ruined relationships with the rest of the family. As mentioned earlier, substance misuse is very common among the young people's biological parents.

The young people have generally not experienced a secure base in their early years where predictability and caring adults were available and often they had no contact with wider family. These findings are also supported by research in other countries (see Cameron et al., 2011; Casas et al., 2010; Höjer et al., 2010; Rácz et al., 2010,). An example of the lack of relationships is illustrated in the following quote from one of the young people interviewed in the study:

> After having been to school, I preferred to be on my own and I still feel that way. It does not bother me. I do not have to be with other people all the time, not at all. I actually prefer to spend time on my own compared to be with others. I can easily be on my own, however, not all the time but because I have always been used to spending so much time on my own, because I had that responsibility, so it has come to be that I do not mind being on my own. I actually have a great need to be on my own. (Nanna)

Nanna draws a connection between her upbringing and her need to be alone. She spent much time on her own as a child because she was responsible for taking care of a younger sister and doing the shopping and cooking. Moreover, the family was isolated and there was no contact with the wider family. So she did not get used to engaging with social communities, which she thinks is why she now prefers to be on her own.

The study has shown that several factors influence the young people's educational pathways. Important positive factors include a stable schooling, supportive parents and carers, early intervention, stability in placement, leisure time activities, social relationships and engaging in social communities. The study showed further that the young people's decision-making and attainment was dependent upon the people in their immediate surroundings. Their environment played an important role as emphasised by one of the interviewed young women identified as belonging to the group of young people on a pathway to college or university:

> I was supported by friends and family who always told me that education was necessary. We discussed what was good and what possibilities you would have after

taking an education. I thought, of course I shall attend upper secondary school, it was a natural step as all my friends also wanted to attend upper secondary school. It would have been abnormal if I had just stopped after compulsory school. (Ditte)

This quote illustrates the positive impact that friends and family can have on the young people's motivation to study since this woman is part of a social community where choices are discussed and supported.

In the next sections, we will focus on social relationships which we have identified as one of the most important factors and are facilitators for the young people to continue their education. We will draw on sociological perspectives in a discussion of individualisation and social relationships in order to discuss why participation in social communities is so important in modern society.

Social relationships and individualisation in modern society

Social relationships and thereby participation in social communities appeared to be very important as the young people had never experienced a secure base/community before coming into care because of the many problems in their families and the many disruptions in their life. Relationships with friends, family and carers were crucial for the young people as these people showed interest, encouraged them and often acted as role models. Gilligan (2007) also highlights the importance of available adults who show interest in the young people's education and provide encouragement. He also stresses that friends in the community and/or family, an attachment person, a social network of peers and positive role models have been identified as providing a variety of resilience-promoting factors (Gilligan, 2001). It is also argued by Stein and Munro (2008) that young people tend to fare better if they are offered stability, opportunities for new attachments, continuity in their relationships with family, carers and friends, and if education is prioritised as part of care planning and where they are well supported when they leave care. Social relationships and social communities were identified in our study as a facilitator throughout the young people's lives. Our study shows that the young people felt that if there was someone to support them in reflecting on choices in life it influenced their motivation to study and to gain qualifications. Otherwise, they were often left to fend for themselves in school; there were no traditions of education in the family and no one to support them, nor did they get substantial support in adult life. Support from the local authorities often stopped when the young people turned 18 years of age.

In the next section, we will discuss why social relationships are so important for young people in care living in modern society by drawing on Giddens (1991), Beck and Beck-Gernsheim (2002) and other researchers with a sociological perspective.

Giddens (1991) argues that, in post-traditional times, we do not worry about the precedents set by previous generations and options are as open as the law and public opinion will allow. All questions of how to behave in society then become matters about which we have to consider and make decisions. Giddens argues that society has become much more reflexive and aware of its own precariously constructed state. As Giddens explains:

> What to do? How to act? Who to be? These are focal questions for everyone living in circumstances of late modernity – and ones which, on some level or another, all of us answer, either discursively or through day-to-day social behaviour. (1991, p. 70)

According to Beck and Beck-Gernsheim (2002), individualisation is a result of modernity where the individual no longer has *any traditions to rely on* and which results in everybody assuming *individual responsibility for choosing and acting.* Katznelson (2004) also confirms in her study that individualisation has gained acceptance at all levels: at the political level, in social policies, in education and labour market policy. These tendencies are captured well in Beck and Beck-Gernsheim's (2002) expression *Individualisation is two folded: risky freedoms.* In a highly individualised society, integration also gives individuals access to vital resources and independent choices. Conditions around integration in individualised society have changed critically with respect to *the social* (Beck & Beck-Gernsheim, 2002).

Bryderup and Frørup (2011) argue that the social aspect should become internalised and form part of an identity, although the individual remains distinctive. Individualisation is, therefore, the story of young people loosening the hold of traditional social and institutional communities, but simultaneously *extending those social networks and communities, which support their choices and actions.* Such a process ensures the development of an identity that is integrated into society and one which continuously gives the young person the opportunity to participate and gain access to vital resources. Bryderup and Frørup (2011) further propose that a focus should be directed towards increasing resources that will enhance the young people's capacity to choose and towards setting up or developing networks that can support these choices.

According to Nielsen and Katznelson (2009), choice in education is influenced by inner and outer oppositions and young people who are not capable of making choices, or like many of those in our study do not have support or informed advice to help them to do so, become 'the reflexive losers of late modernity' (2009, p. 18).

According to Giddens (1991) and Beck and Berk-Gernsheim (2002), there is a demand for young people living in a modern society to be reflexive and make choices. We find that the young people in our study face the dilemmas in modern society. Previously, when tradition dominated, individual actions did not need such in-depth analysis and thought because choices were already prescribed by traditions and customs. The young people in our study do not want to follow their parents' footsteps. They want more in life than their parents and they regard an education as a tool to achieve this goal. On the one hand, they are aware that they have to lead their own life where traditions no longer dominate. On the other hand, analysis shows that they need to be part of social communities in order to live in an individualised world and to avoid becoming the 'reflexive losers of late modernity'. We found that social relationships and social communities are crucial for the young people as they long for acknowledgement and recognition and they need support to be reflexive and make decisions.

Our analysis shows that the young people benefit from social relationships and from being part of social communities established with carers, families and friends but they do not seem to be aware that these social relationships influence their ability to make educational choices. This indicates that the young people to a great extent have internalised individualised thinking. The young people are aware that they need to be responsible for their own life as their pathways are not predetermined by past experiences and they know they cannot rely on help from friends, family or others (Bryderup & Trentel, 2012).

This assertion is reinforced in the stories of the most vulnerable young people in this study, namely the young people with yo-yo pathways in education, those with 'delayed' pathways and the young people with health problems. These three groups had 'fallen behind' their peers in terms of educational qualifications. They are (more than the other groups) lacking support from social relationships with carers, friends and family. Therefore, professionals at all levels must work towards including young people from a public care background in social communities that can offer them a place for reflection, recognition and support in order to develop their social competences (Bryderup, 2010). Individualisation is hence the story of the individuals loosening their ties with traditional social communities, but, paradoxically, individualisation at the same time creates a demand for extending social networks and communities, supporting the young people's choices and actions (Bryderup and Frørup, 2011).

Conclusions

The aim of this research was to explore what facilitates and hinders the educational pathways of young people from a public care background, focusing particularly on social relationships which we have identified as one of the key factors that promote positive educational progression. We have identified five 'ideal types' based on the young people's educational pathways. By comparing these ideal types we found that all the young people were keen to take responsibility and make decisions in life in order to live a different life from that of their parents. However, the extent to which they were able to do this was greatly influenced by their pre-care and in-care experiences. Our findings show that the groups of young people who had social relationships and experienced receiving support from family, carers and friends managed better than the other young people. We can, therefore, conclude that the development of social competences and participation in social communities are of great importance to promote positive educational pathways. Young people who are supported by available and committed parents, or more often carers and friends, are more likely to obtain educational qualifications.

Our empirical data show that the young people are aware that they live in a modern society with no traditions to adhere to. On the one hand, this can be seen as opening up and creating opportunities. On the other hand, it can also be experienced as creating doubt and insecurity because it is the individual who has to take chances and lead his/her own life. The young people in our study know that they have to take responsibility and make their own decisions in life. They have internalised individualised thinking. However, we can also see from their accounts they need support from social relationships and to be part of social communities in order to navigate through life with no traditions to rely on. Social workers and carers need to be much more active in promoting such relationships and encouraging and enabling young people in care to engage in social communities through leisure activities, long-term friendships and preserving contacts with family and former carers.

Notes

[1] The research leading to these results received funding from the European Union's Seventh Framework Programme under grant agreement no. 217297. The research project was undertaken by a team of cross-national researchers from: the Danish School of Education University of Aarhus, Denmark; the Institute for Social Policy and Labour, Hungary; the Research Institute on Quality of Life, University of Gerona, Spain; the Department of Social Work and the Department of Education, University of Gothenburg; and the Thomas Coram Research Unit, Institute of Education, University of London, UK. All the researchers contributed to the research reported here but responsibility for this paper lies with the authors. The views expressed in this paper are those of the authors and not necessarily those of other partners or of the European Union.

[2] Showing educational promise included having completed compulsory school and under-taking further education or just about to start on an education programme. At the age of 19–21 years, all but three of the young people had completed compulsory school. The telephone interviews revealed that 18 young people were studying at the time, 9 were in employment, 3 were unemployed, 1 was on sick benefits, 2 were on maternity leave and 2 chose the category other.

[3] Follow-up interviews were carried out a year after the in-depth interviews.

[4] The young people were asked to nominate an adult that had had a supportive role in their life particularly in relation to education. Sixteen young people nominated an adult, most commonly a foster parent followed by a regular support worker and a grandparent.

[5] See http://tcru.ioe.ac.uk/yippee/ for more information about the whole project.

[6] Invitations to participate in the study were sent to 235 young people but only 75 young people agreed to participate. The 75 young people were drawn from the 5 participating local authorities. The relatively low participation rate may indicate that a lot of young people did not want to discuss their care lives or did not want to be associated with the social services. It may also mean that the young people who agreed to participate in the study are interested in education and, therefore, agreed to participate in the study.

[7] Social relationships are to be understood in a wide sense and include in this study relationships with friends, family, carers as well as the participation in social communities.

[8] It is important to acknowledge that some of the ideal types are based on very small numbers.

[9] See Bryderup and Trentel (2010) for a discussion of all the characteristics.

[10] In this case socio-economic status was an attempt to classify individuals, families and households in terms of indicators such as occupation, income and education. Low

socio-economic status meant that if the parents held a job, it was unskilled and they had no educational qualifications.

References

Andersen, S. H. (red.) (2010). *Når man anbringer et barn – Baggrund, stabilitet i anbringelsen og et videre liv* [When a child is placed in care – Background, stability and future life]. Rockwool Fondens Forskningsenhed og Syddansk Universitetsforlag, Viborg.

Ankestyrelsen. (2009). *Ankestyrelsens statistikker, Børn og ung anbragt uden for hjemmet, kommunale afgørelsen, årsstatisk 2009* [National Social Appeals Board statistics, children and young people in care, decisions, annual statistics 2009]. Author, Odense.

Beck, U. & Beck-Gernsheim, E. (2002) *Individualisation. Institutionalised individualism and its social and political consequences*, Sage, London.

Bryderup, I. M. (2005) *Børnelove og socialpædagogik gennem hundrede år* [Legislations concerning children and social pedagogy through a hundred years], Klim, rhus.

Bryderup, I. M. (2010) *Ungdomskriminalitet, socialpolitik og socialpædagogik* [Youth crime, social policy and social pedagogy], Klim, Aarhus.

Bryderup, I. M. & Frørup, A., (2011) 'Social pedagogy as relational dialogic work – Competences in the modern society', in *Social pedagogy and working with children – A progressive approach.*, ed. C. Cameron, Jessica Kingsley, London, pp. 85–103.

Bryderup, I. M., & Trentel, M. Q. (2010). *Young people from a public care background pathways to education in Denmark*. Retrieved from http://tcru.ioe.ac.uk/yippee/Portals/1/Danish%20report%20-%20WP6.pdf

Bryderup, I. M. & Trentel, M. Q. (2012) *Tidligere anbragte unge og uddannelse* [Young people who have been in care and education], Klim, rhus.

Bryderup, I. M., Trentel, M. Q., & Kring, T. (2010). *WP 3 & 4 – Analysis of quantitative data from Denmark*. Retrieved from http://tcru.ioe.ac.uk/yippee/Portals/1/WP3%20and%204%20-%20Denmark.pdf

Cameron, C., Jackson, S., Hauari, H., & Hollingworth, K. (2011). *Young people from a public care background: Pathways to education in England*. Retrieved from http://tcru.ioe.ac.uk/yippee/Portals/1/WP5report%20UKFINAL%2025.01.11.pdf

Casas, F., Montserrat, C., & Malo, S. (2010). *Young people from a public care background pathways to education in Spain*. Retrieved from http://tcru.ioe.ac.uk/yippee/Portals/1/SpanishWP8.pdf

Christoffersen, M. N. (1993) *Anbragte børns livsforløb. En undersøgelse af tidligere anbragte børn og unge født i 1967* [Children in care pathways. An investigation of children and young people from a public care background born in 1967], Socialforskningsinstituttet, København.

Dixon, J., Wade, J. & Weatherley, H. (2004) *Young people leaving care: A study of outcomes and costs*, Social Work Research and Development Unit, University of York, York.

Egelund, T., Andersen, D., Hestbæk, A., Lautsen, M., Knudsen, L., Fuglsang, R. & Gerstoft, F. (2008) *Anbragte børns udvikling og vilkår* [The development and conditions for children placed outside the home], Socialforskningsinstituttet, København.

Giddens, A. (1991) *Modernity and self-identity, self and society in the late modern age*, Polity Press, Cambridge.

Gilligan, R. (2001) *Promoting resilience: a resource guide on working with children in the care system*, BAAF, London.

Gilligan, R. (2007). 'Adversity, resilience and the educational progress of young people in public Care in': *Emotional and Behavioural Difficulties* 12(2), 135–145.

Glaser, B. & Strauss, A. L. (1967) *The discovery for grounded theory: Strategies for qualitative research*, Aldine de Gruyter, London.

Höjer, I., Johansson, H., Hill, M., Cameron, C., & Jackson, S. (2008). State of the art consolidated literature review. The educational pathways of young people from a public care background in five EU countries. Retrieved from http://tcru.ioe.ac.uk/yippee/Portals/1/Stateothertrevie-woeducationalpathwaysinEuropeFINAL2011.12.08.pdf

Höjer, I., Johansson, H., & Hill, M. (2010). *A long and winding road*. Retrieved from http://tcru.ioe.ac.uk/yippee/Portals/1/Swedishfinalreport.pdf

Jackson, S. & Sachdev, D. (2001) *Better education, better futures: Research, practice and the views of young people in public care*, Barnardo's, Ilford.

Katznelson, N. (2004). *Udsatte unge, aktivering og uddannelse – dømt til individualisering* [Socially disadvantaged young people, activation and education] (PhD Thesis). Roskilde University, Roskilde.

Melbye, J., & Husted, L. (2009). 'Døgnanbragte børn får sjældent en uddannelse [It is uncommon for children in care to get an education]'. In *AKF Nyt no. 2 June 2009* [Danish Institute of Governmental Research news no. 2 June 2009], AKF: København, pp. 6–9.

Mortensøn, M. D. & Neerbek, M. N. (2008) *Fokus på skolegang ved visitation til anbringelse uden for hjemmet. Delrapport 2.* [Focus at schooling in the placement referral], SFI, Copenhagen.

Nielsen, M. L. & Katznelson, N. (2009) *Når fremtiden tegner sig* [The prospekt of the future], Center for ungdomsforskning, København.

Ottosen, M. H. & Christensen, P. S. (2008) *Anbragte børns sundhed og skolegang, udviklingen efter anbringelsesreformen* [Children in care health and schooling, the development after the care reform], SFI, Copenhagen.

Petersen, K. E. (2010) *Viden om anbragte børn og unge i døgntilbud* [Knowledge about children and young people in care], Socialpædagogernes Landsforbund, København.

Petrie, P. & Simon, A. (2006) 'Residential care: Lessons from Europe', in *In care and after: A positive perspective*, eds E. Chase, A. Simon & S. Jackson, Routledge, London, pp. 115–136.

Rácz, A., Csák, R., & Korintus, M. (2010). *Young people from a public care background: Pathways to further and higher education in Hungary*. Retrieved from http://tcru.ioe.ac.uk/yippee/Default.aspx?tabid=398

Stein, M. & Munro, E. (2008) *Young people's transitions from care to adulthood*, Jessica Kingsley, London.

Weber, M. (1949) *Methodology of the social science*, Free Press, Illinois.

Enabling young people with a care background to stay in education in Hungary: accommodation with conditions and support

Gyermekvédelmi gondoskodásban részesülő fiatalok továbbtanulásának segítése Magyarországon: utógondozói ellátás

Andrea Rácz & Márta Korintus

Young people can legally leave care at the age of 18 in Hungary. At that time, they can step out of the child-protection system or have the option of requesting to stay in aftercare provision if they wish to pursue their studies. Aftercare provision is a combination of services that include accommodation, financial support, personal advice, help to find the most suitable form of education, support for studying, assistance to achieve integration into society and conflict management. Most young people choose this option, remain until they are 24 or 25 years of age and become independent roughly at the same age when their peers leave their families to start a life on their own. The article discusses the educational careers of young people with a care background within this context. Children in care are less likely than their counterparts living in birth families to go on with their studies after the compulsory age of completing schooling. Most of them wish to learn some kind of profession, and only a small percentage enter higher education. The system of aftercare provision is a good means to motivate young people in care to study further and to help those who wish to obtain a higher education degree.

Magyarországon a fiatalok ngykorúvá válásuk okán 18 éves kor elérésekor kerülhetnek ki a gyermekvédelmi gondoskodásból. Akkor vagy ténylegesen elhagyhatják a gyermekvédelmi rendszert, vagy az utógondozói ellátást választhatják, ha létfenntartását önállóan biztosítani nem tudják, vagy továbbtanulnak. Az utógondozói ellátás keretében biztosítva van lakhatásuk, pénzbeli támogatást kapnak, személyre szóló tanácsadásban részesülnek, amely a számukra legmegfelelőbb továbbtanulási forma megtalálására is kiterjed, valamint támogatásban részesülnek tanulásukhoz, a társadalomba való beilleszkedéshez és konfliktusok kezeléséhez. A legtöbb gyermekvédelmi gondoskodásban részesülő fiatal ezt a lehetőséget választja és 24 vagy 25 éves koráig a rendszerben marad. Ezáltal többségük ugyanabban az életkorban válik függetlenné, mint amikor a családban nevelkedők kezdenek saját életet. A cikk ebben a kontextusban tekinti át a gyermekvédelmi gondoskodásban részesülő fiatalok továbbtanulását. A gyermekvédelem rendszerében felnövekvő gyermekek kisebb arányban folytatják tanulmányaikat a kötelező tanulmányok befejezése után. Legtöbben valamilyen szakmát kívánnak tanulni, csak kevesen lépnek tovább a felsőoktatásba. Az utógondozói ellátás jó megoldás a fiatalok továbbtanulásának motiválására és a felsőfokú tanulmányokat folytatni kívánók támogatására.

Introduction

We have hardly any information on the life-course of young people leaving public childcare. Policy reports show that, compared with their peers, they rarely continue their studies to higher education (Jackson, 2007). As higher education has become the norm in EU countries, those unable to get a higher qualification will increasingly lag behind and be exposed to risk of social exclusion, as well as to all related disadvantages in terms of health status, employment, income, housing, social participation and attainable life quality. It has therefore become a pressing necessity to keep these young people within the education system.

In Hungary, we have limited information about the educational careers and future perspectives of young people leaving public childcare. Their care is based on social work, whereas the care of children who have not reached the age of legal adulthood is based on pedagogy. Social work-based care work builds on a contractual relationship, where the client and the social worker are equal partners; they agree together on goals and roles in the care process (Rácz, 2009).

The Hungarian system of care for those young people with a care background who continue their studies after the age of 18 is unique because it is a central system, guaranteed and financed by the state, providing complex support. The research project known as YIPPEE, *Young people from a public care background: pathways to education in Europe*,[1] provided an excellent opportunity to look at and discuss the benefits and shortcomings of this system. This article gives a brief introduction to the Hungarian child protection[2] and education systems and then discusses the educational careers of young people with a care background and the role of the aftercare provision in motivating and supporting young people in their further studies.

After-care Provision and Education

The System for Care

During the transition years after 1989, practically all policies related to education, and the protection and support of children and young people, were changed and modernised. The socialist state assumed responsibility for children who lost their parents or were taken out of their families long before the transition. The ideology of socialism, claiming that the state can solve and eliminate all social/societal problems, also meant that children in public care were not considered to be disadvantaged, since the state provided them with secure and suitable care in adequate circumstances. By the 1980s, however, it became evident that the socialist state could not eliminate all situations and factors interfering with children's health development. Consequently, a more permissive attitude towards child protection in Hungary began to make many changes possible. Two major tendencies characterised the changes during the 1980s. First of all, there were the efforts of the workers within the system to change the focus on child protection as a special provision, to one that considers the protection of all children in general. Second, client-centred thinking became more and more widespread, for instance, the idea of family social work emerged (Domszky, 1999). These initiatives did not change the institutional focus of the child-protection system but we can say that the transformation of the child-protection system started earlier than the political changes. The Act 31 of 1997 on the protection of children and guardianship is basically the result of the social historical events of transition.

This Act was accepted by the Hungarian Parliament in April 1997. It is based on the Hungarian Constitution and the Convention on the Rights of the Child, which Hungary signed in 1990. Its importance is highlighted by the fact that this is the first comprehensive, independent legislation concerning child-protection in the history of legislation in Hungary. It re-structured, improved and organised the system of protection for children into a comprehensive whole.

Children's rights and interests are prioritised; therefore, the aim is to bring up children in their own family. The Act is the relevant piece of legislation for all services for children, such as childcare, respite care, residential care and foster care. Using the services is optional. Parents or guardians are required/referred to use them only in certain cases. The two main objectives in relation to children in public care are (1) to help children to get back to live with their own families as soon as possible, and (2) if this is not possible, to promote their integration into society, and to help them achieve an independent life (Rácz et al., 2009).

When reaching the age of 18, young people have the option to leave care or stay within the system if they cannot move back to their families, cannot support themselves and wish to continue their studies. Whatever their decision, when young people leave care after 18, they are eligible for financial support towards buying a home.

If they decide to leave care, they are eligible for *aftercare support* for a minimum of one year, provided that they personally request this. The service is designed to help with leading an independent life through guidance and advice on educational opportunities, labour-market options, financial matters and psychosocial issues.

If they decide to stay in care, *aftercare provision* is available upon the request of young people. It is offered in foster care or in aftercare homes, including accommodation with full provision, personal advice (including legal and financial advice) to start an independent life, advice and support to find the most suitable form of education, support for studying, help to achieve integration into society and conflict management. Young people are eligible in a number of different circumstances: if their short- or long-term care terminated upon reaching legal maturity and they cannot support themselves, or they are in full-time education, if they are a full-time student in higher education, or are waiting for admittance to a social welfare institution. Since 1 January 2010, young adults can apply for aftercare up to the age of 21 if they work or are seeking work, up to the age of 24 if they study; and up to the age of 25 if they are engaged in full-time post-secondary education.

The aim is to support young people until they finish their studies, or until they find a stable job and a suitable living arrangement (Kuslits et al., 2010). Helping young people in care is seen as tertiary prevention, that is preventing their later dependence on social welfare provision (Szikulai, 2004; Kuslits et al., 2010). Successful integration into society for young people with a care background should be considered by taking into account the possibilities and limitations of the care system (Rácz, 2009). It is influenced by several factors such as individual skills and capabilities of children and young people, their level of socialisation, existing resources, personal networks, possible support from family and friends, educational attainment, labour-market position, housing conditions and accessibility of services (Szikulai, 2004). So, though helping those who reach adulthood in care is seen as tertiary prevention, in many cases correctional mechanisms (such as diminishing earlier hospitalisation and schooling disadvantages, restoring family relationships) dominate (Szikulai, 2004; Rácz, 2009). Supporting young people is aimed at developing the knowledge and skills needed for everyday living: shopping, paying bills, handling money, personal hygiene, having a healthy lifestyle, developing and maintaining relationships, taking responsibility for decisions made and accepting the rules of social life (Kuslits et al., 2010).

Child-protection statistics show that the number of children and young adults in care totals 21,468 nationally (0.8% of the general population of children). Roughly half of them live in foster homes and the rest in children's homes or aftercare homes. The number of young people in aftercare provision is 3906. Their placement roughly follows the same pattern. The reason for staying in aftercare provision is the continuation of studies in 67% of cases, not being able to lead an independent life due to the lack of sufficient income in 30% of the cases and waiting to be admitted to a social welfare institution in 3% of the cases (*Gyermekvédelmi statisztikai tájékoztató*, 2011).

Hungarian young people generally leave their families to start an independent life at the age of 25 and a half. Young people in care can stay in aftercare provision until the age of 24 if they study. Most do, so the age of becoming independent is roughly the same for the two groups.

Education

In 1993, the three Acts on public education, higher education and vocational training re-structured the education system and formulated the principles of education on all levels. Among the several modifications in the public education Act, some of the most important ones introduced in 2003 were the prohibition of all kinds of discrimination and the introduction of the rights of children with special educational needs.

Education in Hungary is compulsory between the ages of 6 and 18. Generally, elementary school lasts eight years from age 6 to 14, and secondary education four years from age 14 to 18. To enter tertiary education one must obtain the school leaving certificate ('érettségi') which consists of a series of examinations at the end of secondary school. The school leaving certificate also serves as the entrance examination to higher education. There are three main types of school at secondary level: 'gimnázium' (secondary school), which is part of the normative pathway to tertiary education, 'szakközépiskola' (vocational secondary school), which can also provide the school leaving certificate in addition to an occupational qualification and 'szakmunkásképző' (vocational school) where the main goal is obtaining a job qualification and which does not lead to the school leaving certificate.

Children in care are overrepresented in elementary, vocational and remedial vocational schools, while they are underrepresented in secondary school (gimnázium) and vocational secondary schools, which offer better opportunities for further studies. There are twice as many vocational school students (15.9%), among children living within the child-protection system as in the normal population, and the rate for remedial vocational school students is tenfold (9.4%) (Rácz *et al.*, 2009; Table 1).

Most children placed with foster parents and attending elementary school are in the grade that corresponds to their age, meaning that they did not repeat a grade. The opposite is true for those living in children's homes, where the majority of children are overage for their school class. The indication is that although children living with foster parents are at a disadvantage compared with the national average, they show

Table 1. Number and Proportion of Students in Compulsory Education in Hungary, Year 2007/2008.

Type of school	In Hungary altogether		Those who are in care	
	N	%	N	%
Elementary school	811,405	54.9	7208	67.4
Secondary school	243,152	16.5	251	2.3
Vocational secondary school	281,898	19	516	4.8
Vocational training school	129,066	8.7	1701	15.9
Remedial vocational school	9773	0.7	1013	9.4
Total	1,475,294	100	10,689	100

Source: Oktatási statisztikai évkönyv, 2007/2008 (Hungarian Educational Statistical Guide 2007/2008).

more educational promise than those living in children's homes. Nevertheless, at least one piece of research (Neményi & Messing, 2007) revealed that children's mental abilities influence placement decisions. Those whose development is not delayed have a greater chance of being placed with foster parents. Unfortunately, there is no statistical data or research relating to those in care who enter higher education.

The educational level and labour-market position of parents influence school achievement. Among parents of students living in children's homes, those with a lower-level educational background are overrepresented. Sixty-one per cent of mothers and 53% of fathers have only vocational school, or lower qualifications, whereas the comparable figures among parents of students living with their own families are only 24% for mothers and 18.5% for fathers. There are also significant differences related to the labour-market status of the parents; 65.8% of parents of students living with their own families have a permanent job. This is true for only 50% of birth parents of children in foster placements and 38% of parents of students living in children's homes (Rácz et al., 2009).

School achievement of 15–18 year olds in care who study in vocational school is unfavourable. Thirty-eight per cent failed one or more subjects, and one-third had to repeat a grade in elementary school; 56.9% had to repeat a grade because of low marks. In 22.3% of the cases, family problems had a negative impact on children's achievements. In the school year of 2007/2008, 20% of children in care failed in a subject in vocational secondary school in spite of the fact that roughly the same proportion of these children received personal tutoring as those living with their families. Students who are in care do not think well of their teachers: 60% of them feel that none of the teachers are open to honest personal talks. Their dissatisfaction is manifested in the numerous hours of absence from school. About 20% of them missed more than the accepted maximum of 30 hours (Hodosán & Rácz, 2009).

There is a significant difference regarding plans for future studies: about 41% of students living in care prefer to obtain a vocational training school certificate, whereas this is true for only 11.3% of students living with their own families. On the other hand, 55% of students living with their own families intend to obtain a certificate of higher education, compared with 26% of students living with foster parents and a mere 15% of students living in children's homes. About 6% of those raised in care study in higher education, compared with 21% in the general population (Rácz *et al.*, 2009).

In spite of the high participation rates in vocational schools, the data give no indication of how marketable these qualifications are. One of the eligibility criteria for aftercare provision is if, having reached legal maturity, young people cannot support themselves. Accessing aftercare provision for this reason seems to indicate high unemployment rates and/or ad hoc and illegal jobs among this group. While we could be optimistic that most young people access aftercare provision in order to continue their studies at a higher level, applying for aftercare provision might indicate the motivation only to finish school and/or to obtain another (mostly unmarketable) vocational school certificate (Rácz, 2009). Nevertheless, most young people in aftercare provision stayed within the child-protection system because they wanted to continue to study. They realised that education is the means to get (better) jobs, which are the pre-requisite for leading an independent life.

Based on the data from 'Ifjúság 2008' (Szabó & Bauer, 2009), we can state that in the general population the acquisition of a secondary school leaving certificate does not provide protection against unemployment. Among 15–29 year olds the majority of the unemployed are graduates of elementary school, that is did not continue in education beyond this point (35% unemployed), while 29% of vocational school graduates and 28% of secondary school graduates are unemployed. Unemployment among university graduates however is only 8%.

Educational Career of Young People in After-care Provision

Research Method[3]

Information and data for this discussion paper originate from two sources: national statistics and qualitative data from the EU-funded research, YIPPEE.

The main objective of YIPPEE was to understand how young people's experiences vary in different welfare states in Europe and what action might be taken to improve the educational participation and success of young people from a public care background. The aim of the national studies was to identify and track the progress of 19–21-year olds from a public care background who were still in care at the age of 16 and showed some evidence of 'educational promise'. In Hungary, this term was defined as having passed the secondary school leaving exams (the certificate being the criterion for entering higher education), or taking one of the alternative pathways through the education system to pursue studies, and showing the motivation to continue in further and higher education. Following updating literature reviews and secondary analysis of published statistical data, each national research team conducted a case study in selected areas. These studies consisted of interviews with key policy-makers and service managers and telephone interviews with young people. In Hungary, interviews were carried out with 35 young people, 35 nominated adults in their lives (usually a friend, foster parent or an aftercare provider) and four decision makers. Thirty-four of the 35 young people were interviewed again a year later. The young people interviewed were all staying in aftercare provision and three quarters of them were women. Four of the young people considered themselves of Roma origin. Their average age was 19.5 years. Fifteen of the young people lived with foster parents and 20 in aftercare homes. Ten of them studied in higher education, 8 in secondary school, 11 in vocational school, 1 in vocational secondary school and 5 attended vocational courses.

Educational Experience of Young People

Based on the interviews, four typical educational pathways could be identified (Figure 1). Two of the possible four pathways lead to higher education, and two focus on obtaining vocational qualifications. These pathways become separated at age 14, after primary education, when young people choose which secondary school to attend. The four possible pathways are mapped, starting with secondary-level qualifications:

1. leading to obtaining a profession: vocational school → course(s) → job;
2. leading to obtaining a profession: secondary school leaving certificate (vocational school + two-year additional education programme leading to a secondary school leaving certificate OR vocational secondary school) → course(s) → higher education courses;
3. leading to higher education: secondary school leaving certificate (vocational secondary school, secondary school) → courses, higher education courses → higher education;
4. leading to higher education: secondary school, secondary school leaving certificate → college/university.

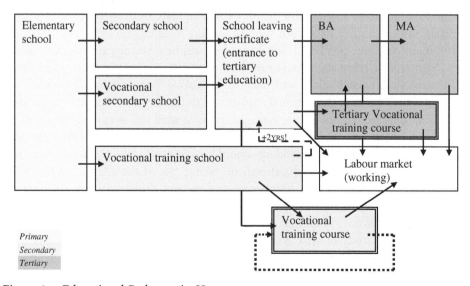

Figure 1. Educational Pathways in Hungary.

The type of secondary school chosen basically determines the available pathways. This primarily concerns those who intend to obtain a vocational qualification by continuing their studies (Pathways 1 and 2). Switching to a pathway that leads to higher education is more difficult for those young people who continued their studies in a vocational school after finishing elementary school, because this type of school does not give the secondary school leaving certificate necessary for entering higher education. It is possible for them to obtain it by completing an extra two-year educational programme. However, this does not frequently happen, because for these young people a secondary school leaving certificate is important only for finding a better job.

The majority of young people raised in care take pathways 1 and 2. This is mainly due to their primary desire to 'stand on their own two feet', i.e. starting an independent, self-reliant life as soon as possible. They believe that the quickest way to achieve this goal is to obtain a vocational qualification. Educators and foster parents working within the child-protection system also regard this as being very important, and tend to believe that only secondary-level qualifications are realistically within the reach of those young people raised in care.

The system of vocational training provided outside the school system is a popular choice of further study for young people in care. These educational programmes last 1–2 years and fit in well with their expectations, since one can obtain a vocational qualification in a relatively short time. Theoretically, each additionally obtained qualification raises the chances of finding a job in the labour market. In the course of these programmes, young people usually do not aim for a qualification that supplements one already obtained. Rather, they learn completely different professions. Typically, young people in care enter such programmes if they fail to progress along the path they had chosen, that is, if they cannot find a job, if they quit school or if they do not get admitted into their chosen higher education institute. They repeatedly go back to one of these programmes after each unsuccessful attempt, and as a result, they obtain several vocational qualifications. For those who already have a secondary school leaving certificate, these programmes provide an alternative to higher education. Several young people complete courses that provide higher level qualifications.

Those young people, who actually make their way into higher education, typically follow pathway 3 or 4. These pathways have a common characteristic: the completion of secondary school gains them a secondary school leaving certificate. Pathway 4 provides a typical, 'straightforward' path towards getting into higher education, and it is predominantly chosen by young people who are not raised within the child-protection system. They usually attend a secondary school and after obtaining the secondary school leaving certificate, they start their higher education studies. Obviously, obstacles and problems can emerge along this pathway, as well. In case of an unsuccessful entrance exam, or a choice of school that proves to be wrong for the young person, pathway 3 presents an alternative. In such cases, young people usually continue their studies by attending courses until they can pass the next entrance exam. Obtaining a job is not a characteristic of these pathways.

The overall majority of the interviewees finished the school grades as expected, but 14 out of the 35 respondents completed secondary school later than the usual age of 18/19. Overall, the majority of the young people interviewed have had positive experiences. Young people feel that professionals working within the child-protection system have a supportive attitude towards school. Many respondents emphasised that learning is regarded as a basic value, together with the principle that everybody is studying for himself/herself. By prioritising the continuation of studies, both foster families and staff working with children and young people enforced the idea that good school performance is the pre-requisite of further successes.

The support received by young people in care may be categorised into (1) support for schoolwork (help with homework assignments, mentoring, tutoring), (2) financing additional costs of studies (financing school supplies, accommodation, travel expenses, the costs of participation in school events) and (3) emotional support (advice, motivation, assistance in career planning).

Young people in care are thankful that their studies are supported, even after they have reached the age of ending compulsory schooling. Support is primarily of a financial nature for those in aftercare homes. In foster homes, there is a greater emphasis placed on emotional support and maintaining personal motivation. It is important to note, though, that the main reason for remaining in the aftercare system after reaching the age of legal maturity is the fact that, in most cases, the young adult has nowhere to go, since she/he has no stable family relationships, so the system provides the only secure place. In many cases, they also take into account the convenience of remaining within the system—since they are provided with accommodation, clothing and support for studies. Furthermore, it is much more economical to stay in the system than to live independently. Those respondents who were committed to studying considered the opportunity for staying in aftercare provision offered within the child-protection system to be especially important for the continuation of their studies.

Supporting Educational Careers After the Age of Ending Compulsory Schooling within the System of Child Protection

Staff and professionals working within the child-protection system consider the preparation of children and young people for an independent life to be their most important mission. This means to prepare them to do everyday chores, to care for and look after themselves and to manage their money. Professionals share the view that realistic goals should be set, which match the needs, capabilities and interests of the children and young people. Supporting young people's decisions is just as important—especially the ones related to pursuing studies and supporting their studies financially. The importance of psychosocial support for children, both at school and in the child-protection system, was emphasised. Some informants believed that there should be fewer children per staff in the child protection institutions so they could be provided with better personalised care.

The support system has several levels. Apart from the immediate help with studies (e.g. with homework), finance, emotional support and encouragement are also provided. On a critical note, however, we should say that childcare professionals do not regard higher-level qualifications as a reachable goal for this target group, so they tend instead to guide them towards obtaining a secondary school leaving certificate and a skilled occupation. They try to protect the young people from failure, even those whose school performance shows that they should, if they were not in care, be heading towards getting a degree.

Hungarian educational policy, unfortunately, does not prioritise targeting young people brought up within the child-protection system. In the opinion of professionals working within the system whom we interviewed there is a need for scholarship programmes for all talented children living in disadvantaged families, not only those in care, and these should be based on well-founded educational and economic policies.

The majority of interviewed professionals highlight the role of schools: the importance of having opportunities for appropriate remedial training, and teachers who have the skills necessary for aiding children in care to solve their problems. Several of them emphasised that the child-protection system needs more professionals, such as developmental teachers, special needs educators and psychologists, and that children need successful examples to serve as role models, for instance through organising programmes and celebrations together with those formerly in care who have become successfully integrated into society.

Conclusions and Discussion

During the transition years after 1989, practically all policies related to education, and the protection and support of children and young people, were changed and modernised. The importance of Act 31 of 1997 is highlighted by the fact that this is the first comprehensive, independent legislation concerning child protection in the history of legislation in Hungary. It re-structured, improved and organised the system of protection for children into a comprehensive whole. This Act is the statutory base for supporting young people until they reach 24 years old (or 25 if they study full time).

We have limited information about the educational careers of young people brought up in the child-protection system. It is known that children in care are less likely than their counterparts living in birth families to go on with their studies after the compulsory age of completing schooling. Only a small proportion enter higher education. Staff and professionals in the child-protection system pay little attention to children pursuing their education, in spite of the general view that studying is important.

Our results show that most of those raised within the child-protection system wish to learn some kind of skill or trade. For many young people growing up in care, starting an independent life as soon as possible is a priority. Typically, educators and foster parents also consider this to be important, and often they consider a secondary certificate as the highest level realistically achievable by these young people. Young adults with a childcare background whom we interviewed usually pursue one of four academic pathways, only two of which lead to higher education, while the other two concentrate on learning a trade.

Young adults, who tend to consider learning and obtaining suitable, competitive qualifications as important, most often highlighted personal ambition, perseverance and will-power as helping them in their studies. However, in their view, a supportive background was also essential. Young people highlighted their financial situation as the most inhibiting factor, many having to contribute to financing their studies—which strains their savings and makes starting an independent life more difficult. Another typical problem is that usually there is not a named, responsible person in the child's life who could help him or her, and childcare institutions have no strategic plans to follow and motivate children in their studies. In the lives of these children, there are no appointed persons who are responsible for their school careers, from the time they are admitted to care until they leave the system forever. Consequently, these children have no real prospects, and they experience difficulties in the course of career planning and future orientation.

It is important to note that significant differences can be found between the academic careers of those studying at graduate and secondary levels; generally, the vast majority of YIPPEE students in higher education had never taken long breaks from their studies—they went straight through secondary school and obtained a certificate.

We saw that the child-protection professionals' attitude to education was considered to be supportive and, by giving priority to studies, the foster family and the children's home confirmed to the young people that good academic performance is a condition for moving forward.

To summarise, we can say that the young adults consider the possibility of using aftercare services to be important, particularly, so that they can study and have extra time for laying the foundations for their future, delaying the transition to fully independent adulthood. Staff and professionals also report that if a young adult wishes to obtain higher education, and this aspiration is considered realistic on the basis of previous school performance, individual ability and motivation, the care system provides every material and moral support.

We have to note, however, that the provisions of the Child Protection Act, implemented on 1 January 2010, have significantly changed the system of aftercare provision. Those unable to sustain themselves (whether working or unemployed) may stay in aftercare accommodation until 21 years of age. Lowering the upper age limit of care to 21 years, without strengthening earlier pedagogical work, poses the danger that precisely those who cannot start an independent life, because of low income or having no income, will leave the system earlier. Systematic pedagogical work with and support for those who apply for after care is also urgent, because there are concerns that these young people, having left the childcare system, will appear in the social welfare system due to their low levels of education, weak labour-market position and small network of connections. Extending care eligibility until 24 years of age exclusively for those in education poses a risk of full-time study becoming preferred because of the associated benefits of accommodation and provision; even when it is not appropriate for the young person's ability and interests.

Recommendations for action to help more young people with a care background to advance to post-compulsory education in Hungary are as follows (Rácz *et al.*, 2011):

1. It is an important requirement that the child's school performance should be documented and followed in a standardised format from the first day of special care. There should be a written plan regarding his or her academic pathway, and there should be a person who takes responsibility for shaping the child's life, and who, thereby, can monitor changes in his or her academic career. This means a shift in approach within child-protection services, creating a focus on planned assistance in academic progress, and preparation for a conscious career choice, in order to lay the foundations of the child's future.

2. Professionals should support qualifications that are suited to the individual's ideas and skills, and foreseeable labour-market demands. It might be useful to set higher expectations (e.g. vocational secondary school and secondary certificate, instead of vocational school), because experience has shown that those who aim for a higher level of education, progress further in the educational system and are more employable.

3. Support for extensive statistical surveys and child protection-related research is necessary in order to gain a deeper insight into the situation of the target group. The present child-protection statistics contain a minimal amount of data on the educational participation of children of compulsory school age within the child-protection system. We have no information whatsoever regarding the level and scope of studies of those who have reached their legal maturity and who are still receiving aftercare provision. Regarding studies in higher education, we only have estimates. A further problem is that data collection is performed at an institutional level, so we do not have child-protection data available at the individual level. Furthermore, the data collected on the education of the overall population do not contain a breakdown for those living within the child-protection system.

4. Continuation of studies after the age of compulsory education is largely determined by whether the children at risk in their families receive all the necessary assistance from childcare to overcome their disadvantages and compensate for failures at school, and whether children who are taken out of their families have access, within the childcare system, to the support necessary

to help them deal with the separation from their families and their familiar environment, and overcome the effects of any traumas that they have experienced.

5. Children living in disadvantaged families and children separated from their families need extensive tutoring and talent-grooming programmes, as well as various fellowships and financial support.

6. It is necessary to strengthen the basic education system, and to prepare teachers to work with children from disadvantaged backgrounds, including those in public care. Child protection and child welfare modules should be incorporated into teacher training.

7. Finally, there should be more attention in schools in ensuring that all children acquire basic skills such as numeracy and literacy, rather than the accumulation of factual knowledge. This is especially important for children in out-of-home care because they are very likely to have missed some of the crucial early stages of schooling due to their disruptive family situations.

Notes

[1]   Funded under the European Union's Seventh Framework Programme under grant agreement no. 217297.

[2]   The term 'child protection' in Hungary encompasses the whole field of child welfare and care and does not simply refer to investigation and intervention in cases of neglect or maltreatment as in the UK usage.

[3]   The research project was undertaken by a team of cross-national researchers from the Danish School of Education University of Aarhus, Denmark; the Institute for Social Policy and Labour (now called National Institute for Family and Social Policy), Hungary; the Research Institute on Quality of Life, University of Gerona, Spain; the Department of Social Work and the Department of Education, University of Gothenburg; and the Thomas Coram Research Unit, Institute of Education, University of London, England. All the researchers contributed to the research reported here, but responsibility for this paper lies with the authors. The views expressed in this paper are those of the authors and not necessarily those of other partners or of the European Union

References

Csécsiné, M. E., Könyvesi, T., Kozma-Lukács, J. & Tuska, Zs. (2008) *Oktatási statisztikai évkönyv, 2007/2008* [Educational Statistical Guide 2007/2008], OKM, Budapest.

Domszky, A. (1999) 'Hol tart a gyermekvédelem?' [How far has child protection progressed?], in *A magyar gyermekvédelmi rendszer helyzete, jövőbeli kihívásai* [Position and future directions of the Hungarian child protection system], ed. A. Rácz, NCSSZI (National Institute for Family and Social Policy), Budapest, digital issue, 2006.

Hodosán, R. & Rácz, A. (2009) 'Szakmai képzésben részesülő, gyermekvédelmi szakellátásban élő fiatalok iskolai pályafutásának vizsgálata' [Educational carriers of children in care who study in vocational schools], *Család, gyermek, ifjúság*, vol. 18, no. 4, pp. 14–24.

Jackson, S. (2007) 'Care leavers, exclusion and access to higher education', in *Multidisciplinary Handbook of Social Exclusion Research*, eds D. Abrams, J. Christian & D. Gordon, Wiley-Blackwell, Chichester, pp. 115–135.

Kuslits, G., Riegler, M. & Rácz, A. (2010) *Utógondozói ellátás protokollja* [Protocol for After-care Provision], Manuscript, SZMI, Budapest.

Neményi, M. & Messing, V. (2007) 'Gyermekvédelem és esélyegyenlőség' [Child protection and equal opportunities], *Kapocs*, vol. 4, no. 1, pp. 2–19.

Nemzeti Család és Szociálpolitikai Intézet—Nemzeti Erőforrás Minisztérium. (2011) '*Gyermekvédelmi statisztikai tájékoztató 2008* [Child Protection Statistical Guide 2008], Nemzeti Család és Szociálpolitikai Intézet-Nemzeti Erőforrás Minisztérium, Budapest.

Rácz, A. (2009) *Barkácsolt életutak, szekvenciális (rendszer)igények—Gyermekvédelmi szakellátásban nevelkedett fiatal felnőttek iskolai pályafutásának, munkaerő-piaci részvételének és jövőképének vizsgálata* [Do-It-Yourself Biographies, Sequential (system)Requirements—Study of the Educational Career, Labour-Market Participation, and Future Perspectives of Young Adults who were Brought Up in the Child Protection System], Unpublished Ph.D. Thesis, University of Eötvös Lóránt, Institute of Sociology and Welfare Policy.

Rácz, A., Hodosán, R. & Korintus, M. (2009) 'Dokumentumok, szakirodalmak a gyermekvédelmi rendszerben élő, fiatal felnőttek továbbtanulásáról és felsőoktatási részvételéről' [Literature review on access to further and higher education among young people from public care backgrounds], *Esély*, vol. 3, pp. 97–114.

Rácz, A., Csák, R. & Korintus, M. (2011) *Secondary Analysis of National Data Sets and Survey of A Sample of Child Care Agencies in Hungary—A Case Study*, Institute for Social Policy and Labour, Budapest, [Online] Available at: http://tcru.ioe.ac.uk/yippee/Default.aspx?tabid=398

Szabó, A. & Bauer, B. (eds) (2009) *Ifjúság 2008—Gyorsjelentés* [*Youth 2008*], SZMI, Budapest.

Szikulai, I. (2004) *A nagykorúvá váltak gondozásának módszerei* [Care Methods for Young Adult]. in *Gyermekvédelmi szakellátás*, ed. A. Domszky, NCSSZI, Budapest, pp. 267–274.

Placement, protective and risk factors in the educational success of young people in care: cross-sectional and longitudinal analyses

Des facteurs de placement, de protection, et de risque dans le succès scolaire des jeunes placés: Analyses transversales et longitudinales

Robert J. Flynn, Nicholas G. Tessier & Daniel Coulombe

In the present study, we formulated and tested a basic model of the educational success of young people in out-of-home care. We used data from 2007 to 2008 and 2008 to 2009 on a sample of 1106 young people in care in Ontario, Canada. The youths were 12–17 years of age; 56.24% were male and 43.76% female. The indicators of educational success in both years were the youth's average marks and the youth's school performance in reading, math, science and overall, as rated by his or her caregiver. Based on resilience theory and on a model of the influence of maltreatment on educational achievement, our model included four categories of predictors: control variables (youth gender and age and, in the longitudinal analyses, the year 7 value of the year 8 dependent variable), three placement types (foster, kinship care or group homes), three risk factors (previous repetition of a grade in school, a health-related cognitive impairment index and a measure of behavioural difficulties) and three protective factors (caregiver involvement in the youth's school, caregiver educational aspirations for the young person and the youth's total number of internal developmental assets). Cross-sectional and longitudinal hierarchical regression analyses provided mixed support for the proposed model. The youth's gender, level of behavioural difficulties and number of developmental assets, and the caregiver's educational aspirations for the young person, emerged as the most consistent predictors of educational success. The implications and limitations of the findings were discussed.

Dans cette étude, nous avons formulé et évalué un modèle de base du succès scolaire des jeunes qui ont été placés en dehors de leur famille d'origine. Nous avons utilisé des données dont la saisie s'est faite en 2007–2008 et 2008–2009 auprès d'un échantillon composé de 1106 jeunes placés dans la province d'Ontario au Canada. L'âge des jeunes étaient entre 12 et 17 ans; 56.24% étaient de sexe masculin et 43.76% de sexe féminin. Les indicateurs du succès éducatif chaque année étaient la moyenne des notes scolaires du jeune ainsi que sa performance en lecture, mathématiques, science, et dans l'ensemble des matières. Notre modèle, basé sur la théorie de la résilience ainsi que sur un modèle de l'influence de la maltraitance sur le rendement scolaire, incluait quatre catégories de prédicteurs : des variables de contrôle statistique (le sexe et l'âge et, dans les analyses longitudinales, la valeur dans l'an 7 de la variable formant la variable dépendante dans l'an 8), trois types de placement (des familles d'accueil, des familles de parenté, et des foyers de groupe), trois facteurs de risque (le fait d'avoir redoublé à l'école, un indice composé de plusieurs difficultés cognitives reliées à la santé, et un indice des difficultés du jeune sur le plan du comportement), et trois facteurs protecteurs (l'implication du parent d'accueil dans la vie de l'école du jeune, les aspirations du parent d'accueil envers le jeune, et le nombre total des acquis internes de développement du jeune). Des analyses de régression transversales et longitudinales ont fourni un soutien partiel au modèle proposé. Le sexe, le niveau de difficultés de comportement, le nombre d'acquis de développement, et les aspirations du parent d'accueil envers le jeune se sont révélés les meilleurs prédicteurs du succès éducatif. Les implications ainsi que les limites des résultats ont été explorés.

Introduction

Many young people in out-of-home care (hereafter, 'in care') in Europe, North America and other regions experience educational difficulties, including cognitive deficits, poor problem-solving and reasoning skills, inconsistent school attendance, below-average academic performance and low scores on standardised tests of academic achievement in reading, writing and mathematics (Flynn *et al.*, 2004;

Jackson, 2007; Slade & Wissow, 2007; Trout *et al.*, 2008). In the USA, Trout *et al.* (2008) conducted a comprehensive review of the American educational research conducted on young people in care and published in journals during the period of 1940–2006. The 29 studies reviewed described the academic status of a total of 13,401 young people in care; they had a mean age of 12.9 years, and 52% were male. On the whole, the young people in care had a much higher level of risks in school functioning than the general youth population, with frequent changes in schools and high levels of grade retention, suspension and school dropout. The young people in care were nearly three times as likely to be involved in special education as their age peers in the general population, tended to score in the low to low-average range on measures of academic achievement, and were often rated by their teachers as academically at risk. Trout *et al.* (2008) suggested that many youths in care presented academic deficits similar to those identified in reviews of the academic status of other at-risk populations, including children with emotional and behavioural disorders and maltreated children who had been reported to child welfare agencies.

In the UK, Jackson (2007) reviewed the progress made over the last 20 years in improving the educational outcomes of young people in care. She found that considerably better data on their academic status now existed and that coordination had improved between local educational and child welfare services. In addition, the issue of education for children in care had risen to the top of the policy agenda, with local authorities now required to promote their educational attainment. Berridge (2007) noted that there was recent evidence of a slight improvement in outcomes in the UK. The proportion of young people in care obtaining one General Certificate of Secondary Education (GCSE) or equivalent had increased from 53% to 60% between 2002 and 2005, but this improved level of achievement was still much lower than the level of 96% on the same criterion in the general child population. Moreover, the proportion of young people in care who had obtained five or more GCSEs had increased only from 8% to 11% during 2002–2005, whereas in the general population the level had increased from 52% to 56%.

Jackson (2007) agreed with Berridge (2007) that there had been little attempt in the UK to understand the basic reasons for the achievement gap, while disagreeing with his view that the answer lay in the characteristics of the families of origin of children in care rather than in weaknesses of the care system itself. Jackson (2007) suggested that discussions of foster parent recruitment and selection had largely ignored the large body of research that identified a strong link between children's academic performance and the educational level and expectations of their parents or caregivers. She added that the problem in the UK of ensuring an adequate education for young people in the care system also characterised the child welfare systems of other English-speaking countries. This appears to be true for Australia (Cashmore *et al.*, 2007) and the USA (Trout *et al.*, 2008), and also, as we shall see, of Canada. The educational attainment gap also appears to characterise other countries, however, such as Sweden (Vinnerljung *et al.*, 2005) and Norway (Iversen *et al.*, 2010). Weyts (2004), cited in Iversen *et al.* (2010), for example, found that the reading skills of

Norwegian children in care were no better than those of children in care in England, the Netherlands and Spain.

In Canada, the relatively few studies conducted to date on the educational achievement of young people in care provide a sketch similar to the portrait in the countries previously mentioned. In the province of Ontario, Flynn and Biro (1998) found that children in care had higher rates of grade retention and school suspension than their age peers in the general population. Flynn *et al.* (2004) compared the ratings made by caregivers in Ontario of the educational performance of children and adolescents in their care with the ratings made by parents in the general Canadian population of their own children's educational progress. Eighty per cent of the young people in care aged 10–15 years and 78% of the children in care aged 5–9 years were rated by their foster parents as performing in the same range as the lowest third of the children in the general population, who had been rated by their parents on the same composite measure of reading, spelling, math and overall educational performance.

In more recent research in Ontario, Miller *et al.* (2008) pointed to some possible reasons for the achievement gap. Sixty-eight per cent of the young people in care aged 10–15 years in their sample had changed schools three or more times for reasons unrelated to normal progression through the school system, and the percentage repeating a grade was 16% among 5–9 year olds in care, 27% among 10–15 year olds and 32% among 16–20 year olds.

In Ontario, as elsewhere, academic difficulties seem especially prevalent among boys in care. Miller *et al.* (2009) found that girls in care were less likely than boys to undergo assessments for learning-related problems (58% vs. 79%) or to receive special academic help at school (49% vs. 69%). Caregivers also rated the girls' school performance more highly: 24% of the girls were rated as performing 'Very Well' or 'Well' in written work, compared with 13% of the boys; 41% of the girls (vs. 28% of the boys) were seen as doing 'Very Well' or 'Well' in reading; and 29% of the girls (vs. 20%) were rated as doing 'Very Well' or 'Well' overall. Only in math were equal proportions of boys (23%) and girls (24%) rated as performing 'Very Well' or 'Well'. The girls also tended to be more positive about education-related matters than the boys: 37% (vs. 28%) said, for example, that they read 'for fun' every day, and 40% (vs. 26%) aspired to attain one or more university degrees.

Recently, the Ontario Association of Children's Aid Societies (OACAS, 2010), in collaboration with 43 of its local member agencies, carried out a review of the files of 4694 Crown Wards or former Crown Wards (i.e., young people in relatively long-term out-of-home care). The youths were 16–20 years of age and had been in school during 2008–2009. OACAS compared the results from 2008 to 2009 with those from a similar study conducted in 2006–2007. The results showed that the youths in care had results that fell well short of those of their age peers in the general population, although some progress had been made in the two-year interval since the initial study. The percentage of 16 and 17 year olds not attending any educational programme (Ontario requires school attendance up to age 18) had declined from 14% to 7%. Graduation from secondary school had increased by 2%, from 42% to

44%, compared, however, with a larger increase in the general youth population, from 75% to 79%. The number of former Crown Wards aged 18–20 who were enrolled in post-secondary education (PSE) had increased from 21% to 23%, compared to 39% in the general population. Of those in PSE, 81% were now in community colleges, including apprenticeship programmes (vs. 84% two years earlier), compared with 19% in university (vs. 16% two years earlier).

The purpose of the present study was to formulate and test a basic model of educational success among young people in care that included the standard control variables of gender and age and selected placement, protective and risk factors. In formulating the model, we were guided by two theoretical frameworks. First, we drew upon Masten's (2006) conceptualisation of resilience theory: 'Resilience refers to positive patterns of functioning or development during or following exposure to adversity, or, more simply, to good adaptation in a context of risk' (p. 4). Masten (2006) noted that 'Direct predictors of better outcomes often are described as *assets* or *resources*' (p. 6). As predictors of academic achievement, good examples of assets would be high-quality parenting or higher IQ scores. In the risk-related child-welfare context of providing care for formerly abused or neglected young people, assets may be called *protective factors* because they appear to play an especially important role in positive adaptation. *Risk factors*, on the other hand, are predictors of undesired outcomes. In the context of educational performance, abusive or neglectful parenting or severe poverty would be good examples. Masten (2006) suggested that a typical 'short list' of factors associated with resilience in children and youth includes *relationships and parenting* (e.g., strong links with one or more effective parental figures; high-quality parenting that provides affection, monitoring and expectations); *individual differences* (e.g., learning and problem-solving skills; self-control of attention, emotional arousal and impulses); and *community context* (e.g., effective schools; positive organisations).

Second, we used the framework proposed by Slade and Wissow (2007), in which maltreatment is hypothesised as influencing educational outcomes through two main pathways. The first pathway consists of mental health problems stemming from abuse or neglect, including disruptive classroom behaviours, suspensions or difficulties of concentration and motivation. The second pathway comprises inadequate cognitive stimulation at home, lower-quality informal and formal education, and poorly developed academic skills in word knowledge, literacy and numerical reasoning. Slade and Wissow (2007) further hypothesise that the maltreated youth's mental health difficulties and low academic skills raise his or her risk of not adhering to behavioural norms at school, obtaining less support from teachers and classmates, doing poorly on homework assignments and tests and ultimately performing inadequately in school.

In the present study, we defined *educational success* in terms of two outcomes: the youth's *average marks* during the last year in school, and his or her *school performance* as rated by the caregiver on a composite measure of reading, math, science and overall performance. Based on the literature reviewed, we included four categories of predictors in our basic model of educational success. The first category consisted of the standard control variables of gender and age, although we also saw female gender as a protective factor because of girls' greater educational success than boys (Miller *et al.*, 2009). Regarding age, we had no expectation that older youths would perform any better or worse than younger youths. The second category of predictors, corresponding to Masten's (2006) 'community context' factor, comprised the type of placement in which the young person had been living, whether a foster home, kinship care home or group home. In line with McClung and Gayle's (2010) findings regarding the role of placement type, we anticipated that youths living in smaller settings (i.e., foster or kinship care homes) would succeed better in school than those residing in larger settings (i.e., group homes). The third category of predictors consisted of three risk factors that we believed would be negatively associated with educational success: having previously repeated a grade in school (Flynn & Biro, 1998), a lower level of cognitive functioning (Masten, 2006) and a higher level of behavioural difficulties (Slade and Wissow, 2007). The fourth category of predictors comprised three protective factors suggested by Masten's emphasis on the key role of assets or resources in promoting better adaptation. Two parenting-related assets were, respectively, a greater degree of involvement by the parental figure (caregiver) with the young person's school, and a higher level of aspirations on the part of the caregiver regarding the young person's eventual level of educational attainment. The third resource was the young person's level of internal developmental assets, chosen because of prior evidence that a greater number of developmental assets is associated with greater educational success both in the general population (Scales *et al.*, 2006) and in young people in care (Flynn & Tessier, 2011).

Method

Participants and Service Context

The sample consisted of 1106 young people in care, aged 12–17; 56.24% were male and 43.76% female. The young people had participated in both year 7 (2007–2008) and year 8 (2008–2009) of the Ontario Looking after Children (OnLAC) project (Flynn *et al.*, 2006; Flynn *et al.*, 2009), which annually monitors the service needs and developmental outcomes of children and youth who have been in care for a year or more in the province. The OnLAC project is mandated by the provincial government in local Children's Aid Societies (CASs) across Ontario to encourage more data-based decision-making about children's needs, improve the quality of the substitute parenting they receive and enhance their short-term and long-term outcomes.

At the time the data were gathered, child welfare services in Ontario were provided or supervised by a network of 53 government-funded CASs, the number of which was beginning to be reduced through amalgamations in a search for greater efficiency and sustainability. There were approximately 18,500 children and youths in out-of-home care, over half of whom were teenagers (Commission to Promote

Sustainable Child Welfare, 2010). Excluding older youths in supported transitional or independent living, 80% of the days of care provided in Ontario in 2009–2010 were spent in family-based care (i.e., family foster care or kinship care), 15% in group care and 5% in other settings (e.g., hospitals, youth justice settings or children's mental health settings). Approximately 40% of expenditures in child welfare in Ontario were allocated to in-care services (Commission to Promote Sustainable Child Welfare, 2010).

Instrument

The child welfare worker responsible for a given young person in care administered the data collection instrument from which all the measures in the present study were taken, namely, the second Canadian adaptation of the Assessment and Action Record from Looking after Children (AAR-C2-2006; Flynn *et al.*, 2009). The AAR-C2-2006 consists of eight age-appropriate formats, each of which comprises a family of instruments. Administration of the tool is done annually, in the form of a structured conversational interview in which the young person in care (if aged 10 or over), his or her caregiver and his or her child welfare worker take part. The information gathered in the AAR-C2-2006 interview is used to carry out a major revision, each year, of the young person's plan of care for the ensuing 12 months.

The AAR-C2-2006 consists of questions that cover nine areas: a background section, completed mainly by the child welfare worker, that provides basic descriptive information on the young person, caregiver and child welfare worker; seven sections, rated mainly by the young person in care and his or her caregiver, that assess the youth's service needs and developmental outcomes in each of the Looking After Children domains, namely, health, education, identity, social and family relation-ships, social presentation, emotional and behavioural development and self-care skills; and a final section, adapted from the work of the Search Institute (Scales *et al.*, 2000), in which the child welfare worker rates the young person's acquisition of 40 different developmental assets (Flynn *et al.*, 2009).

Criterion (Outcome) Measures

Two criterion measures of educational success were selected from the year 7 AAR-C2-2006 data for the eventual cross-sectional analyses, and the same two measures were taken from the year 8 data for the longitudinal analyses. The first measure was the *average marks* that the young person in care had attained during the previous year in school or during the last year he or she had been enrolled in school. The possible values were 4 (<50%), 5 (51–60%), 6 (61–70%), 7 (71–80%), 8 (81–90%) or 9 (90–100%). The second measure was the young person's *school performance,* as assessed by the caregiver on a four-item composite scale consisting of ratings of how well the youth had done in school in years 7 and 8 on language and reading, mathematics, science and overall. Each item was rated on a 3-point scale: 0 = Very

Poor or Poor; 1 = Average; and 2 = Very Well or Well. The total score on school performance could range from zero to eight.

Predictor Measures
Control variables
Female gender was assigned the value of one and *male gender* the value of zero. The young person's *age* was his or her age in years as of the date that the AAR-C2-2006 interview had begun in OnLAC year 7.

Placement type
Three dichotomous variables were used to represent the type of placement setting in which the young person in care had resided in OnLAC year 7: Foster Home (1 = Yes, 0 = Other), Kinship Care Home (1 = Yes, 0 = Other) or Group Home (1 = Yes, 0 = Other). In the regression analyses, the group home dichotomy served as the reference category and was thus omitted.

Risk-factor measures
The measures of the three risk factors were taken from the AAR-C2-2006. The first was a dichotomy that indicated whether the young person in care had *ever repeated a grade in school* (1 = Yes, 0 = No). The child welfare worker provided this information, with assistance, as needed, from the caregiver and young person. The second risk-factor measure was a health-related *Cognitive Impairments Index* that we created. The index consisted of the youth's total number of cognitively related long-term health conditions (out of a maximum of four), as rated by the youth's child welfare worker. These health conditions had lasted or been expected to last for 6 months or more, had been diagnosed by a health professional, and, by their very nature, were likely to pose a challenge to the youth's cognitive functioning. The child welfare worker indicated which of the following health conditions the youth had: Learning Disability (1 = Yes, 0 = No), Developmental Disability (1 = Yes, 0 = No), Attention-Deficit Disorder (1 = Yes, 0 = No) and Fetal Alcohol Syndrome (1 = Yes, 0 = No). The score on the index could range from zero to four.

The third risk-factor measure was the youth's score on the *Total Difficulties Scale* of the Strengths and Difficulties Questionnaire (SDQ; Goodman, 1997), which is embedded in the AAR-C2-2006. The SDQ Total Difficulties Scale, composed of 20 behavioural items rated by the caregiver (0 = Not True, 1 = Somewhat True and 2 = True), covers the domains of emotional symptoms, conduct problems, hyperactivity/inattention and peer problems. The total score could range between 0 and 40.

Protective-factor measures
The three protective-factor measures were also taken from the AAR-C2-2006. The first two were educationally relevant aspects of high-quality parenting on the part of the caregiver. The *Caregiver School Involvement Index* consisted of the number of

school activities (out of a maximum of eight) in which the caregiver reported having been involved during the current or last school year, such as volunteering in the young person's class or attending a school event in which the young person had participated. The second protective-factor measure, *Caregiver Aspirations,* consisted of the caregiver's expressed hope that the young person in care would achieve a certain level of education (1 = Primary or elementary school; 2 = Secondary or high school; 3 = Trade, technical, vocational school or business college; 4 = Community college or nursing school; 5 = University).

The third protective-factor measure consisted of the number of *Internal Developmental Assets* (out of a maximum of 20) possessed by the young person in care. The 20 asset items were rated by the youth's child welfare worker (1 = Yes, 0 = Uncertain or No). The internal assets covered four areas: the youth's commitment to learning (e.g., 'The young person is motivated to do well in school'); the young person's positive values (e.g., 'The young person accepts and takes personal responsibility'); the youth's social competencies (e.g., 'The young person knows how to plan ahead and make choices'); and the young person's positive identity (e.g., 'The young person feels that he/she has control over "things that happen to me"').

Data Analysis
Preliminary analyses
We began by assessing whether we would need to conduct multi-level analyses of our data, in which the young people in care would be nested within their respective local CASs. We found that this would not be necessary, as the amount of overall variance accounted for by CASs in our two measures of educational success was very small and statistically non-significant. We also evaluated whether we would need to control for the particular geographic region (out of a total of six) in Ontario within which the youth's CASs was located. This, too, turned out to be unnecessary, as geographic region was not significantly related to either measure of educational success.

Hierarchical regression analyses
We related our two criteria of educational success, average marks and school performance, to the four categories of predictors (controls, placement type, risk factors and protective factors), in a series of hierarchical regression analyses. Two cross-sectional analyses were conducted, in which the year 7 outcomes served as the dependent variables. Similarly, two longitudinal analyses were carried out, in which the year 8 outcomes were the dependent variables and in which the year 7 values of the criterion variables were entered as control variables in step 1 (along with gender and age). These longitudinal analyses tested the ability of our predictive models to account for *change* from year 7 to year 8 in the two educational outcomes.

Results

Descriptive Results

Paired t-tests (not shown) revealed that, on the outcome of young people's average marks, there was no significant mean change from year 7 ($M = 6.54$, $SD = 1.01$) to year 8 ($M = 6.56$, $SD = 1.04$; $t(784) = 0.29$, $p = 0.77$). There was also no change on the other outcome, school performance, between year 7 ($M = 4.21$, $SD = 2.37$) and year 8 ($M = 4.32$, $SD = 2.26$; $t(857) = 1.42$, $p = 0.16$).

Table 1 presents basic descriptive information on the study variables. On some, the effective sample size was < 1106 because, for example, some young people were in ungraded classrooms and thus had no data on the outcome of average marks. Other youths were in placement settings that were neither foster, kinship, nor group homes, such as mental health or juvenile justice residential settings and were eliminated from the analyses. On other variables, the caregiver or child welfare worker were uncertain about the young person's previous scholastic history (e.g., regarding whether the young person had previously repeated a grade).

Over half of the young people (52.1%) had no health-related cognitive impairments, whereas 29.1% had only one, 13.7% had two, 4.3% had three and 0.8% had the maximum of four. The internal consistency coefficients (Cronbach's alphas) for four of the multi-item measures were excellent, in the 0.80s. On our two constructed indexes, internal consistency was lower. It was acceptable (0.62) in the case of the eight-item Caregiver Involvement in School Index but marginal on the

Table 1 Means (or percentages), standard deviations and Cronbach's alphas for study variables

Variable	N	Mean (or %)	SD	Cronbach's Alpha
Outcomes				
Average marks—Year 7	894	6.51	1.03	–
Average marks—Year 8	878	6.54	1.03	–
School performance in Year 7	975	4.11	2.39	0.89
School performance in Year 8	942	4.28	2.27	0.88
Control variables				
Gender (1 = Female, 0 = Male)	1106	43.76%	–	–
Age (in years)	1106	13.99	1.34	–
Placement type				
Foster home (1 = Yes, 0 = Other)	1058	72.40%	–	–
Kinship care home (1 = Yes, 0 = Other)	1058	7.09%	–	–
Group home (1 = Yes, 0 = Other)	1058	20.51%	–	–
Risk factors				
Previously repeated a grade (1 = Yes; 0 = No)	825	20.73%	–	–
Cognitive impairment index	1106	0.73	0.91	0.45
SDQ total difficulties	1045	12.64	7.44	0.87
Protective factors				
Caregiver involvement in school	902	3.10	1.67	0.62
Caregiver aspirations	855	3.79	1.01	–
Internal developmental assets	1106	12.75	5.10	0.88

brief Cognitive Impairments Index (Cronbach's alpha $= 0.45$). Despite this, the latter correlated significantly and in the expected direction with virtually all of the other variables (see Table 2).

Predictors of Educational Success
Inter-correlations

Table 2 showed, as anticipated, that the four measures of educational success were positively and significantly inter-correlated. Other findings were also as expected: the girls had better outcomes than the boys in both years; all 12 of the correlations between the risk factors and outcomes were negative and statistically significant, and 10 of the 12 correlations between the protective factors and outcomes were positive and significant. On the other hand, the correlations between the three types of homes with the educational outcomes were weak, although in the expected direction, and only half were statistically significant.

Hierarchical Regressions
Average marks

Table 3 displays the results for the cross-sectional (left-hand panel) and longitudinal (right-hand panel) regression models for the outcome of average marks. In the cross-sectional model, the control (step 1), risk (step 3) and protective factors (step 4) all accounted for statistically significant increments in the amount of variance accounted for in year 7 average marks, and there was a trend in the same direction in the case of the placement types (step 2).

The cross-sectional model as a whole accounted for 20.5% of the variance in year 7 average marks, with the risk and protective factors together explaining 17.2%. As predicted, youths in the foster and kinship care homes had higher average marks than those in group homes (step 2), although the relationship was modest. Once the three risk factors had been entered into the model, however (at step 3), the beta coefficients for the placement types were reduced to nearly zero, indicating that their association with educational success was probably mediated by the risk factors. In the final model (at step 4), the youth's total number of internal developmental assets was the strongest predictor of average marks. Caregiver aspirations and youth behavioural difficulties were also statistically significant predictors, and there was a trend in this direction in the instance of female gender and previous repetition of a grade in school.

As previously noted, there was no significant mean change in the youths' average marks between year 7 and year 8. Thus, it was not surprising that the longitudinal model explained little additional variance in year 8 average marks, once the role of year 7 average marks and female gender (which was associated with improved marks at all four steps) had been taken into account. Only two additional predictors—the caregiver's level of involvement in school activities and the youth's level of internal developmental assets—were significantly associated with year 8 average marks.

Table 2 Inter-correlation matrix

Variables	1.	2.	3.	4.	5.	6.	7.	8.	9.	10.	11.	12.	13.	14.	15.
1. Average marks—Year 7	—														
2. Average marks—Year 8	43***	—													
3. School performance—Year 7	64***	35***	—												
4. School performance — Year 8	37***	60***	48***	—											
5. Gender (1 = F, 0 = M)	13***	18***	13***	13***	—										
6. Age (in years)	−01	−03	00	−07*	02	—									
7. Foster home (1 = Y, 0 = N)	01	04	07*	04	10***	−09**	—								
8. Kinship care home (1 = Y; 0 = N)	04	08*	07*	06	02	−02	−45***	—							
9. Group home (1 = Y, 0 = N)	−04	−11**	−13***	−09**	−13***	11***	−82***	−14***	—						
10. Previously repeated a grade (1 = Y; 0 = N)	−10*	−10*	−13***	−13***	−04	−00	04	−06	−00	—					
11. Cognitive impairment index	−11***	−12***	−23***	−19***	−20***	−10***	−02	−12***	10**	13***	—				
12. SDQ total difficulties	−27***	−19***	−37***	−24***	−10***	−01	−18***	−12***	27***	08*	31***	—			
13. Caregiver involvement	10**	16***	03	05	−01	−22***	−03	01	03	08*	11***	04	—		
14. Caregiver aspirations	26***	16***	35***	28***	15***	−06	07*	06	−13***	−13***	−34***	−29***	03	—	
15. Internal developmental assets	34***	28***	43***	33***	18***	−06*	21***	11***	−30***	−06	−24***	−54***	07*	29***	—

Note: Decimals omitted in correlations. Correlations are pair-wise; the number of cases on which the correlations were based varied between 652 (for the correlation between *Previously Repeated a Grade* and *Caregiver Aspirations*) and 1106.
* p < 0.05 (2-tailed); ** p < 0.01 (2-tailed); *** p < 0.001 (2-tailed).

Table 3 Beta coefficients in hierarchical regressions of average marks on control, placement, risk and protective variables

Outcome variable: Average marks in Year 7 Cross-sectional regression (β) (N=531)					Outcome variable: Average marks in Year 8 Longitudinal regression (β) (N=488)				
Predictors	Step 1	Step 2	Step 3	Step 4	Predictors	Step 1	Step 2	Step 3	Step 4
					Average marks (Year 7)	0.42***	0.42***	0.40***	0.37***
Female gender	0.15***	0.14*	0.11**	0.07†	Female gender	0.14***	0.14***	0.12**	0.11**
Age	−0.03	−0.02	−0.05	−0.02	Age	−0.02	−0.02	−0.03	−0.00
Foster home		0.10†	0.01	−0.04	Foster home		−0.00	−0.02	−0.03
Kinship care home		0.11*	0.03	0.02	Kinship care home		0.05	0.03	0.03
Previously repeated a grade			−0.11*	−0.08†	Previously repeated a grade			−0.02	−0.03
Cognitive impairments index			−0.04	0.00	Cognitive impairments index			−0.07	−0.07
SDQ total difficulties			−0.28***	−0.13*	SDQ total difficulties			−0.02	0.02
Caregiver involvement in school				0.03	Caregiver involvement in school				0.10*
Caregiver aspirations				0.18***	Caregiver aspirations				0.02
Internal developmental assets				0.25***	Internal developmental assets				0.10*
ΔR^2	0.024*	0.009†	0.095**	0.077**	ΔR^2	0.214***	0.003	0.006	0.018**

Note: $^*p < 0.05$ (2-tailed); $^{**}p < 0.01$ (2-tailed); $^{***}p < 0.001$ (2-tailed); $^†p < 0.10$ (2-tailed).

School performance

Table 4 shows the results for the two models for school performance. In the cross-sectional model, the results were similar to those for average marks. The control, risk and protective factors all accounted for statistically significant increments in the variance, and the findings for step 2 were at the level of a trend. The cross-sectional model as a whole explained 28.2% of the variance in year 7 school performance, with the risk factor of behavioural difficulties especially important as a predictor. The foster and kinship care homes were again modestly associated with better school performance, but their beta coefficients were reduced to near zero once the three risk factors (all of which were significantly and negatively associated with school performance) had entered the model. In the final model, at step 4, the risk factor of behavioural difficulties and the protective factors of caregiver aspirations and youth internal developmental assets were all significantly related to school performance.

In the longitudinal analyses, the lack of significant change in year-to-year school performance meant that the model had relatively little power to predict change in year 8 school performance, once year 7 school performance had been taken into account. Interestingly, the girls had relatively consistent improved school performance, at all four steps, whereas the older youths had fairly consistent worse performance, at all four steps. In the final model (at step 4), caregiver aspirations for the youth's educational attainment was the only protective factor that was significantly associated with better school performance.

Discussion

The findings provide some, albeit mixed, support for our basic model of educational success and have implications for improving the educational success of young people in care. First, in the cross-sectional regression model for average marks (i.e., in year 7), all four steps in the regression model were associated with increments in the amount of variance accounted for, either at statistically significant levels (steps 1, 3 and 4) or at the level of a trend (step 2). The risk (9.5%) and protective factors (7.7%) explained important proportions of the variance in average marks. Similarly, with respect to school performance, statistically significant increments in the variance accounted for were also found at steps 1, 2 and 4, and a trend in this direction was seen at step 2, with the risk (17.4%) and protective factors (8.3%) accounting for important increments in the amount of variance explained in school performance. The fact that in the longitudinal analyses steps 2–4 accounted for much less additional variance in the two outcomes was no doubt due to the fact that, on average, there was little or no change to explain.

Second, the girls in our sample, as predicted, experienced greater educational success than the boys, on both outcomes. The sequential reductions in the size of the beta coefficient for female gender at each step of the mode, especially pronounced in the cross-sectional models, suggested that the girls' educational advantage was partly

Table 4 Beta coefficients in hierarchical regressions of school performance on control, placement, risk and protective variables

Outcome variable: school performance in Year 7 Cross-sectional regression (β) (N=565)					Outcome variable: school performance in Year 8 Longitudinal regression (β) (N=518)				
Predictors	Step 1	Step 2	Step 3	Step 4	Predictors	Step 1	Step 2	Step 3	Step 4
					School Performance (Year 7)	0.42***	0.42***	0.37***	0.33***
Female gender	0.12**	0.12**	0.06	0.02	Female gender	0.10*	0.10*	0.09*	0.08†
Age	0.02	−0.02	−0.00	0.03	Age	−0.08*	−0.08*	−0.09*	−0.07†
Foster home		0.09†	−0.02	−0.06	Foster home		−0.02	−0.05	−0.06
Kinship care home		0.11*	−0.00	−0.02	Kinship care home		0.04	0.01	0.01
Previously repeated grade			−0.11**	−0.08*	Previously repeated a grade			−0.04	−0.03
Cognitive impairments index			−0.11*	−0.04	Cognitive impairments index			−0.05	−0.03
SDQ total difficulties			−0.37***	−0.22***	SDQ total difficulties			−0.09†	−0.05
Caregiver involvement in school				0.03	Caregiver involvement in school				0.04
Caregiver aspirations				0.23***	Caregiver aspirations				0.10*
Internal developmental assets				0.21***	Internal developmental assets				0.06
ΔR^2	0.016*	0.009†	0.174***	0.083***	ΔR^2	0.200***	0.003	0.012†	0.012*

Note: $^*p<0.05$ (2-tailed); $^{**}p<0.01$ (2-tailed); $^{***}p<0.001$; (2-tailed); $^†p<0.10$ (2-tailed).

mediated by lower levels of the risk factors and higher levels of the protective factors. Despite this, the girls' educational advantage tended to persist even after the risk and protective factors had been introduced into the model.

Third, age had no relationship to educational success, in three of the four regression models. In the fourth, however, age was consistently and negatively associated with improved school performance, indicating perhaps that older youths tend to fall further behind as the academic curriculum becomes more demanding.

Fourth, we found, as expected, that young people in foster and kinship care homes had better educational outcomes than those in group homes, at least in the cross-sectional models. This advantage was modest, however, and disappeared when the risk factors had been taken into account. This was probably due to mediation and may reflect a selection rather than a programme effect, with more turbulent youths being selected out of foster or kinship care and into group care.

Fifth, it is clear that young people in care—of both genders—would benefit from lower levels of behavioural difficulties. The cross-sectional results for this latter variable were congruent with Slade and Wissow's (2007) hypothesis that poor behavioural skills have a serious negative impact on the educational success of maltreated youth. Previous repetition of a grade in school was also predictive of lower educational success in the cross-sectional models, even when the youth's level of health-related cognitive functioning had been taken into account. This indicated that effective action to prevent young people from repeating a grade is likely to pay dividends.

Sixth, in all four models, the protective factors were associated with a statistically significant increment in the amount of variance explained in the two indicators of educational success. The young person's level of internal developmental assets was particularly important for educational success (except in the case of improved school performance), which is congruent with the findings of Scales *et al.* (2006).

Seventh, it was noteworthy that caregiver attitudes and behaviour were related to both indicators of educational success. Higher educational aspirations on the part of caregivers were associated with better outcomes in three of the four regression models, and caregiver involvement in a greater number of school activities predicted significant improvement in the youth's average marks. These results are consistent with Jackson and Ajayi's (2007) position that caregivers are an important resource for improving educational outcomes and should be recognised as such. The recruitment and training of carers should thus take explicit account of their influential role in the educational achievement of young people in care (Dill *et al.*, 2012; Ferguson & Wolkow, 2012; Jackson & Cameron, 2012).

The present study had a number of limitations. The data were correlational in nature, and the longitudinal analyses covered only a 12 month period. Also, the effective sample size was considerably reduced due to incomplete data on some variables. In addition, our index of health-related cognitive impairment was a rather rudimentary measure of current cognitive functioning, and our measure of caregiver aspirations for the young person in care was but a single item. Despite these limitations, our analyses were based on relatively large samples and employed comprehensive measures of two important predictors, the risk factor of behavioural difficulties and the protective factor of internal developmental assets. In future, with the accumulation of large samples and additional longitudinal data, we plan to carry out multi-year analyses of the educational trajectories of subgroups of young people in care, in the hope of identifying those in particular need of intervention. As Trout *et al.* (2008) commented, many young people in care appear to need intensive and effective assistance, if their educational careers are to be as successful as possible.

Acknowledgements

We gratefully acknowledge the financial support of this study by the Ontario Association of Children's Aid Societies and the Ontario Ministry of Children and Youth Services. We also thank the many young people in care, caregivers and child welfare workers in local Children's Aid Societies who participated in the Ontario Looking After Children project, from which the study data were drawn.

References

Berridge, D. (2007) 'Theory and explanation in child welfare: Education and looked after children', *Child and Family Social Work*, vol. 12, no. 1, pp. 1–10.

Cashmore, J., Paxman, M. & Townsend, M. (2007) 'The educational outcomes of young people 4–5 years after leaving care: An Australian perspective', *Adoption and Fostering*, vol. 31, no. 1, pp. 50–61.

Commission to Promote Sustainable Child Welfare. (2010, December) *Future directions for in-care services in a sustainable child welfare system*, Working paper no. 3, Toronto, ON, Commission to Promote Sustainable Child Welfare.

Dill, K., Flynn, R. J., Hollingshead, M. & Fernandes, A. (2012) 'Improving the educational achievement of young people in out-of-home care', *Children and Youth Services Review*, vol. 34, pp. 1081–1083. doi:10.1016/j.childyouth.2012.01.031

Ferguson, H. B. & Wolkow, K. (2012) 'Educating children and youth in care: A review of barriers to school progress and strategies for change', *Children and Youth Services Review*, vol. 34, pp. 1143–1149. doi:10.1016/j.childyouth.2012.01.034

Flynn, R. J. & Biro, C. (1998) Comparing developmental outcomes for children in care with those of other children in Canada. *Children and Society*, vol. 12, pp. 228–233.

Flynn, R. J. & Tessier, N. G. (2011) 'Promotive and risk factors as predictors of educational outcomes in supported transitional living: Extended care and maintenance in Ontario, Canada', *Children and Youth Services Review*, vol. 33, pp. 2498–2503.

Flynn, R. J., Dudding, P. M. & Barber, J. G. (eds) (2006) *Promoting Resilience in Child Welfare*, Ottawa, ON, University of Ottawa Press.

Flynn, R. J., Ghazal, H., Legault, L., Vandermeulen, G. & Petrick, S. (2004) 'Use of population measures and norms to identify resilient outcomes in young people in care: An exploratory study', *Child and Family Social Work*, vol. 9, pp. 65–79.

Flynn, R. J., Vincent, C. & Legault, L. (2009) *User's Manual for the AAR-C2-2006*, Ottawa, ON, Centre for Research on Educational and Community Services, University of Ottawa.

Goodman, R. (1997) 'The strengths and difficulties questionnaire: A research note', *Journal of Child Psychology and Psychiatry*, vol. 38, pp. 581–586.

Iversen, A. C., Hetland, H., Havik, T. & Stormark, K. M. (2010) 'Learning difficulties and academic competence among children in contact with the child welfare sytem', *Child and Family Social Work*, vol. 15, pp. 307–314.

Jackson, S. (2007) 'Progress at last?', *Adoption and Fostering*, vol. 31, no. 1, pp. 3–5.

Jackson, S. & Ajayi, S. (2007) 'Foster care and higher education', *Adoption and Fostering*, vol. 31, no. 1, pp. 62–72.

Jackson, S. & Cameron, C. (2012) 'Leaving care: Looking ahead and aiming higher', *Children and Youth Services Review*, vol. 34, pp. 1107–1114.

Masten, A. S. (2006) 'Promoting resilience in development: A general framework for systems of care', in *Promoting Resilience in Child Welfare*, eds R. J. Flynn, P. M. Dudding & J. G. Barber, Ottawa, ON, University of Ottawa Press, pp. 3–17.

McClung, M. & Gayle, V. (2010) 'Exploring the care effects of multiple factors on the educational achievement of children looked after at home and away from home: An investigation of two Scottish local authorities', *Child and Family Social Work*, vol. 15, pp. 409–431.

Miller, M., Flynn, R. & Vandermeulen, G. (2008) *Looking After Children in Ontario: Good Parenting, Good Outcomes: Ontario Provincial Report (Year Six)*, Reports for 0–4, 5–9, 10–15, and 16–20 year olds, Ottawa, ON, Centre for Research on Educational and Community Services, University of Ottawa.

Miller, M., Vincent, C. & Flynn, R. (2009) *Looking After Children in Ontario: Good Parenting, Good Outcomes. Ontario Provincial Report (Year Seven)*, Report for 10–15 year olds, Ottawa, ON, Centre for Research on Educational and Community Services, University of Ottawa.

Ontario Association of Children's Aid Societies (OACAS). (2010) *Gateway To Success: Cycle Two*, OACAS survey of the educational attainment of Crown Wards and former Crown Wards, ages 16 through 20, during the 2008–2009 academic year, Toronto, ON, Ontario Association of Children's Aid Societies.

Scales, P. C., Benson, P. L., Leffert, N. & Blyth, D. A. (2000) 'Contribution of developmental assets to the prediction of thriving among adolescents', *Applied Developmental Science*, vol. 4, pp. 27–46.

Scales, P. C., Benson, P. L., Roehlkparain, E. C., Sesma, A. & van Dulmen, M. (2006) 'The role of developmental assets in predicting academic achievement: A longitudinal study', *Journal of Adolescence*, vol. 29, pp. 691–708.

Slade, E. P. & Wissow, L. S. (2007) 'The influence of childhood maltreatment on adolescents' academic performance', *Economics of Education Review*, vol. 26, pp. 604–614.

Trout, A. L., Hagaman, J., Casey, K., Reid, R. & Epstein, M. H. (2008) 'The academic status of children and youth in out-of-home care: A review of the literature', *Children and Youth Services Review*, vol. 30, pp. 979–994.

Vinnerljung, B., Öman, M. & Gunnarson, T. (2005) 'Educational attainment of former child welfare clients: A Swedish national cohort study', *International Journal of Social Welfare*, vol. 14, pp. 265–276.

Weyts, A. (2004) 'The educational achievements of looked after children: Do welfare systems make a difference?', *Adoption and Fostering*, vol. 28, no. 3, pp. 7–19.

Addressing low attainment of children in public care: the Scottish experience

Graham Connelly & Judy Furnivall

Policy and practice in relation to the education of looked-after children in Scotland have been significantly influenced as a result of two landmark reports, Learning with Care and Looked After Children: We Can and Must do Better. This paper provides an account of the main policy developments which are set within the distinctive Scottish legal and educational context. The second report, in particular, has been followed by a more strategic approach to implementing change. There is evidence of considerable infrastructural development, both in the looked-after children sector and more widely in education services. There is also evidence of improvement in outcomes, notably in school attendance and the attainment of children in out of home care. While outcomes generally still lag behind those of children who are not looked after, those of children who are looked after while remaining in the family home remain relatively resistant to improvement. This aspect has been neglected in research so far. It is also not well understood how the policy changes have impacted on organisational change and developments in practice.

Introduction

The education of children in public care has been given particular attention by national and local government in Scotland since deficiencies in provision were first identified by an inspection report in 2001 (Her Majesty's Inspectors of Schools and Social Work Services Inspectorate, 2001). This paper provides an explanatory account of the main policy developments in the past decade within the broader context of improving opportunities for looked-after children.

Scotland has always been different from the rest of the UK in relation to education and children's services as a result of its distinctive legal and education systems, and the distinctiveness of these institutions has been important in developing Scotland's approaches to social welfare provision. The law in Scotland developed separately from the law in England and Wales, at least until 1707. Scots law has retained differences because of its different origins, although there are aspects of law which are identical throughout the UK, such as the statutes relating to benefits. Following the introduction in 1999 of devolved government in the UK, distinctive approaches have emerged in policy areas affecting children and families. The Scottish Parliament has the authority to make law in relation to devolved matters and a considerable number of acts and related statutory instruments which affect education and children's welfare services have come into force, of which important examples are the Adoption and Children (Scotland) Act 2007, the Looked after Children (Scotland) Regulations 2009, and the Getting it Right for Every Child guidance (Guthrie, 2011; Scottish Government 2011c).

In Scotland, children in public care, or 'looked-after' children, are principally those for whom the state provides compulsory measures of 'supervision' as defined by the Children (Scotland) Act 1995, though some children become looked after under voluntary agreements. Compulsory measures are actions taken for the 'protection, guidance, treatment or control' of children under a set of conditions (e.g. lack of parental care, failure to attend school regularly, committing an offence) specified in Section 52 (2) of the Act. In Scotland, in 2010, almost 16,000 children were in the care of the state (Scottish Government, 2011a). This figure accounted for 1.4% of all children up to age 18 across the country, although the proportions of children in state care are higher in the larger cities (e.g. 2.8% in Glasgow). The process of becoming looked after involves a children's hearing, at which a panel of three volunteer members of the community considers background reports and listens to the views of the child, family members and professionals. If the panel concludes that compulsory measures of care are necessary it will specify whether these should be provided 'at home', i.e. with the child remaining in the usual family home (40% of all looked-after children) or 'away from home'. Half of all children looked after away from home live in family-type settings, either with trained foster carers or potential adoptive parents, or in so-called 'kinship' settings where a member of the close or extended family is officially recognised as the main carer. A minority (10%) of looked-after children is cared for in group settings, including residential homes in the community (also called 'units', young people's centres or children's houses), residential schools and secure care settings. This figure is an average, however, and when age is taken into account it is evident that foster care is more common as a placement for younger children and residential care for older children. For example, 20% of 12–15 year-old looked-after children live in residential settings, compared with less than 3% of 5–11 year-olds and a negligible proportion of under fives. The overall proportion of looked-after children cared for in group settings has been falling over a period of many years in comparison with increasing proportions of children living in foster and kinship placements. For example, in 1976, 36% of looked-after children lived in residential settings, and only 22% were in foster care.

Evidence of low attainment by children in public care and the related lack of attention to education by professionals were first highlighted in England by Jackson (1987). The concerns have since become a significant aspect of public policy within the different UK administrations (Department of Education and Skills, 2007; Department of Health Social Services and Public Safety Northern Ireland, 2007; Scottish Executive, 2007; Welsh Assembly Government, 2007). Indeed these are matters of concern throughout Europe, notably in relation to the perceived role of education in breaking the intergenerational transmission of poverty, since it is typically children at risk of poverty who are also at risk of becoming looked after by public agencies (European Commission, 2008, 2009).

It was some years before the concerns raised by Jackson began to influence research and policy development in Scotland, although, once begun, the attention of academics, policy-makers and practitioners was quickly mobilised. The rapid pace of development was probably a function of a combination of the small country effect, the prominence given to education and children's services within devolved government and the significant development of civil servant capacity since 1999. The origins of specifically Scottish interests in the education of children in care—a group now referred to as 'looked-after children'—came with the publication of a study highlighting a tendency to concentrate on behaviour rather than academic performance in childcare reviews (Francis *et al.*, 1996) and of a review of research, policy and practice (Borland *et al.*, 1998).

Two government reports are key markers of policy and practice development. The first reported on the inspection of the education of 50 children in residential care settings in five of Scotland's 32 local authorities (Her Majesty's Inspectors of Schools and Social Work Services Inspectorate, 2001; Maclean and Gunion, 2003). The *Learning with Care* report contained nine recommendations, such as the advice that 'local authorities should develop an integrated policy covering education and social work which ensures that the educational needs of looked-after children are met effectively' (p. 34).

The second report, *Looked After Children & Young People: We Can and Must do Better*, was published six years later when the issue of the education of children in care settings had become a matter of significant political concern and a substantial knowledge base had been developing as a result of the dissemination of guidance for practice, professional training, conferences, seminars and research (Scottish Executive, 2007). The report's 19 actions emphasised the crucial link between well-being and success in education and had four distinctive features. First, it was published by the government itself, rather than by a quasi-governmental body, and consequently had greater authority. Second, it was framed to emphasise the rights of looked-after children to the same prospects envisaged for all of Scotland's children, and therefore the concerns about education and attainment were set within broader parameters of well-being and aspiration. Third, it was concerned with looked-after children in all settings, in contrast to the earlier report's focus solely on children in residential care. This aspect was significant for the report's capacity to influence policy and practice, since around 40% of Scotland's 16,000 looked-after children receive support whilst remaining in the family home. Fourth, the report adopted, for the first time in an official document in Scotland, the concept of 'corporate parent' a term encapsulating the obligations of local authorities sharing the parenting of looked-after children. Both reports will be considered further later in this paper.

Concerns about the well-being of looked-after children in Scotland are set within a broader social policy context which while being interpreted for the legal and cultural characteristics of Scotland derive from contemporary international aspirations for improving rights and social justice for children (UN General Assembly, 1989; Scottish Executive, 1999; Gudbrandson, 2007). These aspirations include defining and extending citizenship rights, combating social exclusion, tackling inequalities and seeking to overcome barriers to accessing services. In relation to the educational opportunities and attainment of disadvantaged groups, the discourse of social justice which encompasses concepts, such as values, life-skills and empowerment, is particularly relevant (Hoskins, 2008).

This paper, therefore, argues that the conditions for improving services for looked-after children, particularly in respect of their rights to a good education and better prospects in post-school education and employment, have been considerably advanced by several aspects of policy and practice change. Three particular aspects—the origins of government intervention, the developing policy landscape and the training of workers—are discussed in this paper, and these are related to the educational outcomes of looked-after children.

The Origins of Government Intervention

The *Learning with Care* report was arguably successful in three particular ways. First, it pinpointed significant weaknesses in relation to the support in education for children who had been removed from the family home with the aim of improving their welfare. For example, statutory care plans were found to be of varying quality, or were missing; they typically included little useful information about education, and were not routinely shared with schools. These deficiencies were also found in a later file audit of care plans (Vincent, 2004). Second, through its recommendations, the report highlighted features of good practice. Third, it set in train a sequence of policy and practice reforms which are continuing 10 years later. For example, one of the recommendations called for 'joint professional development for education and social work staff and carers' (p. 34) and this resulted in the *Learning With Care: Improving Outcomes for Looked After Children Project*. The project produced a range of products including training materials, a report based on consultations with children in care about their educational experiences (Ritchie, 2003), an information booklet aimed at carers, social workers and teachers (Connelly *et al.*, 2003) and a set of quality indicators designed to be used within the general framework of school self-evaluation[1] but aimed at all partners in children's services (Her Majesty's Inspectorate of Schools, 2003). The process of development of these materials has been outlined in more detail elsewhere (Connelly, 2003; Furnivall and Hudson, 2003).

Another example of government intervention led to an attempt to provide cash support directly to children in out of home care. A total of £10 million was paid to local authorities, based on the allocation of £500 per child looked after 'in a family home' and £2500 for each child in residential homes, schools and secure accommodation (Scottish Executive, 2001). The intention of the fund was to influence attainment by providing books, computer equipment and homework materials. As a strategy it was somewhat naive. While the additional funding was welcomed, there were also criticisms of the approach for being short term, rushed and non-sustaining. A report prepared by the charity Who Cares? Scotland indicated that of 170 young people surveyed, 98 (58%) were unaware that money had been invested in their education and few had been given a say in the spending (Boyce, 2004).

As a result of such criticism, the publication of the 2007 report, *Looked After Children & Young People: We Can and Must do Better*, was followed by the establishment of a high-level committee sitting during 2007–2008, and short-life working groups, to oversee the implementation of the report's recommendations. This strategic approach to influencing change was more effective and the government established a further strategic planning group which began working in the autumn of 2010. A review of Scotland's residential childcare services (the National Residential Child Care Initiative) proposed time-limited 'activity hubs' to take forward recommendations in respect of workforce development, commissioning of services and physical and mental health (Bayes, 2009). While accepting the review's main recommendations, the government broadened the scope of implementation to encompass the needs of looked-after children living in all settings, and also to give the 'hubs'—care planning, workforce commissioning, improving health outcomes and improving learning outcomes—more status and a definitive strategic planning role by establishing a high-level governance group which has adopted an open approach to its work by making its working papers publicly available.[2]

The Developing Policy Landscape

The policy landscape in relation to the education of looked-after children in Scotland can be characterised by two types of output: the first type is the reports or guidance documents which are specifically dedicated to the task of outlining the needs of looked-after children and good professional practice; the second type is the documents not exclusively concerned with looked-after children but which have incorporated the needs of looked-after children into their content.

In the first category are policy documents concerned with education and achievement; additionally, there are documents concerned with health needs, though these are not discussed here. The report, *Looked After Children & Young People: We*

Can and Must do Better, identified the problems and made proposals for improvements (Scottish Executive, 2007). There are two particular features of the report which are noteworthy. The first is its uncompromising tone, evident in the choice of title, the explicitness with which the actions are stated and the rather unusual inclusion of paragraphs within the report's sections giving the Ministerial working group's reactions to the evidence presented to them:

> Thus the group was shocked at how highly looked after children and young people feature in the exclusion rates from school. They felt that whilst it is important that head teachers retain the right to exclude disruptive pupils, schools also need to be aware of the many challenges and obstacles looked after children and young people face; schools need to deal with looked after children and young people's behaviour in, and attitudes to, school with sensitivity. (Scottish Executive, 2007, p. 23)

The second began life as a simple cosmetic feature, but has come to have significant utility. The government's printers used a blue, green and pink colour scheme with a distinctive spiral motif on the cover and this design was subsequently used to identify all documents emanating from the Scottish Government Looked After Children Unit. This was a deliberate action to make the materials instantly recognisable and more easily accessible, and also to encourage inter-professional collaboration by using a neutral brand which was not associated with a single professional group.

Detailed guidance on the responsibilities of agencies sharing parental responsibilities is provided in *These are our Bairns*[3]: *A Guide for Community Planning Partnerships on being a Good Corporate Parent* (Scottish Government, 2008c). This policy guide introduces the notion of the wider 'corporate family' and 14 of its 17 chapters outline actions and outcome measures for services.

The schools' inspectorate report, *Count Us In: Improving the Education of Looked After Children,* part of a series of reports dealing with different aspects of inclusive education, was based on fieldwork in 15 local authorities, with the specific aims of investigating provision for children at risk of missing out on education and identifying good practice and barriers to progress (Her Majesty's Inspectorate of Education, 2008). The report highlighted teachers' lack of awareness of which pupils were looked after, and ineffective systems for tracking children and their attainment, particularly in the case of those receiving services while living in the family home. The inspectors reported positively on progress made in relation to the development of integrated policies on looked-after children involving education and social work agencies, and on the provision of professional development opportunities for staff. The report was followed by the publication of a tool for evaluating services for looked-after children, *How Good is Our Corporate Parenting*, which makes clear that local authorities have obligations to evaluate the quality of the educational environment that goes beyond the school and into the placement setting (Her Majesty's Inspectorate of Education, 2009).

The practice guide, *Core Tasks for Designated Managers in Educational and Residential Establishments in Scotland* (Scottish Government, 2008a), details the responsibilities of corporate parents in respect of education, identifying 27 'core tasks'. Two important features of the guide demonstrate how thinking about policy in relation to looked-after children has progressed in Scotland since 2003. First, guidance was provided for the entire spectrum of education, from early years to further and higher education. Second, the designated manager role was extended to encompass residential children's homes and residential schools.

Despite the increasing amount of attention given to addressing the educational needs of looked-after children, researchers have highlighted deficiencies in data collection, particularly in relation to attainment and in longer term tracking of the progress of individual children (Jackson and Martin, 1998; Jacklin *et al.*, 2006; Connelly *et al.*, 2008; Brodie, 2010). *The Educational Outcomes of Scotland's Looked After Children and Young People: A New Reporting Framework* introduced changes in the method of data collection (Scottish Government, 2009c). The reporting period shifted from the financial year to the academic year to permit more accurate comparisons to be made between looked-after children and non-looked-after children; previously data reported have been based on a census of children looked after on a single date, 31 March. Future reports will also include only those children who have been looked after for the entire academic year. The second change made provision for the use of a unique reference number to help improve the accuracy of data collection. This device should allow a greater degree of monitoring, with the possibility of longitudinal tracking of the progress of cohorts of looked-after children for research and of individual children for professional purposes. A third, but more problematic, potential change relates to the desirability of sharing data collected by different agencies (e.g. education, social services, health and children's hearings), a matter of much concern to politicians (Scottish Parliament Public Audit Committee, 2011).

Earlier in this paper a distinction was made between policy outputs which are exclusively about looked-after children and those which have incorporated the needs of looked-after children into their content. Two examples of the latter are presented because of their potential importance for influencing practice.

The Education (Additional Support for Learning) (Scotland) Act 2009 amended the law in respect of school placing requests for children with additional support needs in education. One provision gave legal force to the presumption that looked-after children should have 'additional support' in relation to their education:

> ... a child or young person has additional support needs if the child or young person is looked after by a local authority. (within the meaning of section 17(6) of the Children (Scotland) Act 1995 (c36))

The result is that there is an entitlement to assessment of additional support needs where a child or young person is looked after by the state. This entitlement is spelled out in a new code of practice for professionals, *Supporting Children's Learning* (Scottish Government, 2010b):

In discharging their responsibilities towards looked after children and young people authorities are obliged to take steps to consider the educational progress of these children and young people. These steps should include establishing whether looked after children and young people require additional support to enable them to benefit from school education and which of those with additional support needs meet the requirements for having a co-ordinated support plan. (p. 14)[4]

The proponents of statutory intervention argued that too often looked-after children did not receive appropriate support for their education (Francis, 2008). This view prevailed but a contrary view has been voiced by some practitioners who argue that it is wasteful of resources to prove additional supports are not required in the case of looked-after children apparently coping well in school. The education inspectorate indicated that the additional support needs of looked-after children continued to be inconsistently addressed, particularly in the case of children looked after at home and in kinship care (Her Majesty's Inspectorate of Education, 2010).

The second example is *Included, Engaged and Involved: A Positive Approach to Managing School Exclusions* which provides detailed information, covering six pages, about looked-after children, the impact of exclusion on their lives, advice about avoidance of exclusion and the procedures which must be followed if exclusion is judged to be unavoidable (Scottish Government, 2011b). The previous advice on exclusion, issued in 2003, included only a single sentence about looked-after children and the tenor of the guidance put the decision-making power almost exclusively in the hands of the school. This simple metric is evidence of the extent to which the rights of looked-after children to receive a consistent schooling have become recognised within the broader educational community.

The Training of Workers

Looked After Children & Young People: We Can and Must do Better gave a commitment to improve opportunities for access to training for parents, foster carers, residential workers, teachers—including teachers in training—social workers and health workers. Training for professionals, particularly inter-disciplinary training, had begun as a result of the recommendations of *Learning with Care* (Her Majesty's Inspectors of Schools and Social Work Services Inspectorate, 2001). The 2007 report provided an opportunity to reinforce messages about training needs and to take advantage of advances in educational technology. Therefore, multi-media training materials, which included a specially commissioned film, *Craig's Story*, dramatising the effects on education of a young child becoming looked after as a result of neglect and abuse, were developed and produced in DVD-ROM format (Furnivall *et al.*, 2008). The interactive DVD was designed for individual study or for use in courses, and several course options were provided, including a short briefing seminar and a full three-day course.

More than 20,000 copies of the DVD were distributed within children's services during 2008–2009, for example, to every educational establishment in Scotland, from nurseries to universities and approximately 200 staff were briefed as trainers to cascade training sessions within local authorities and other agencies. An information leaflet for teachers and related professionals was prepared to support training and was hosted on the website of the teachers' registration body, the General Teaching Council for Scotland, an illustration of cooperation between institutions aimed at raising awareness (Scottish Government, 2008b).

In a further example of inter-agency collaboration, a national looked-after children website was created, provided as a micro-site located within the main website of the national curriculum support agency, Learning and Teaching Scotland. The aim of the website is to provide a portal to information, guidance, reports and good practice examples for relevant professionals, carers and parents, with linkage to the support materials in the main website, including those in another micro-site, ParentZone. References to 'parents' in this area were changed to the more inclusive wording, 'parents and carers'.

The *Learning with Care* report had advocated that residential children's homes should aspire to be educationally rich environments:

> As part of their quality assurance procedures local authorities should undertake an audit of their residential units to assess how far they are educationally rich environments and, where shortcomings are found, make plans to take appropriate action. (Her Majesty's Inspectors of Schools and Social Work Services Inspectorate, 2001)

The concept of the educationally rich environment is useful in countering un-stimulating intellectual conditions and low educational expectations of looked-after children, barriers to attainment which have been highlighted by many observers over the years (Berridge, 1985; Kahan, 1994; Berridge and Brodie, 1998; Jackson and McParlin, 2006). The dissemination of information about looked-after children, in all settings, particularly about their additional support needs in education, as well as further training for designated managers and other children's services' professionals with specialist roles, provides the basis for improvement and there is compelling evidence that focusing on education can be effective in improving outcomes (Gallagher *et al.*, 2004; Centre for Excellence and Outcomes in Children's Services, 2008; Brodie, 2010). Raising awareness among workers has been mirrored by care standards,[5] drawing attention to the rights of children to receive good educational experiences and have adequate study facilities, including access to computers and the Internet.

Is there Evidence of Improvement?

The preceding sections of this paper have presented evidence in support of the proposition that policy and governance innovations have demonstrated the serious intentions of politicians and children's services' professionals to improve the educational outcomes for looked-after children in Scotland. This is clearly a long-term commitment and improvements in attainment, access to post-school education and employment prospects cannot be expected to follow immediately, or dramatically. Also, official statistics tell only part of the story, since they cannot communicate the experiences of individual children and their carers and teachers. They tend to emphasise inadequacies and also to hide the achievements of looked-after children which may take longer to develop and in many cases will have taken more circuitous paths than those of more advantaged children (Happer *et al.*, 2006; Duncalf, 2010). Nevertheless, statistics are useful in pointing to trends and highlighting concerns. This section of the paper, therefore, examines information published in government statistical reports in respect of the education of looked-after children and considers whether these provide evidence that efforts in policy development and awareness raising are beginning to make an impact on standard outcome measures.

School Attendance

Unsurprisingly, there is a positive relationship between attendance at school and attainment, shown, for example, in a large-scale study of schools in Ohio, USA (Roby, 2004). Looked-after children in Scotland had almost twice the average number of absences from school in 2008–2009 as those not looked after: 45.0 half days compared with 25.0 (Scottish Government, 2009a). But it is the absence from school of children looked after 'at home' (average number of half days' absence = 58.7) which accounts significantly for the poor overall outcome, while children looked after in out of home care settings (residential, foster and kinship care) have absences only a little higher than their non-looked-after peers (28.1 half days compared with 25.0). Table 1 shows the percentage attendance at school of looked-after children during the period 2003–2004 to 2009–2010, compiled from official Scottish Government annual reports. What is evident is the considerable improvement in attendance of children looked after in out of home care settings, while those looked after at home continue to have significantly poorer attendance at school. It seems reasonable to conclude that carers are as effective as the parents of non-looked-after children at ensuring that children attend school.

Exclusion from School

The rate at which they are excluded from school provides an indication of the disruption of education experienced by some looked-after children. Students can be excluded from school for behaviour regarded as unacceptable, following a formal procedure. The most common reasons for exclusion are 'general or persistent disobedience' and 'verbal abuse of staff', accounting for 58% of all cases of temporary exclusions in 2008/2009 (Scottish Government, 2010c). Most exclusion occurs for short periods of up to three days before the student returns to the same school, though some are considerably longer. Table 2 shows temporary exclusions of looked-after children in Scotland over a seven-year period.

Table 1. Attendance of Looked-after Children: 2003–2004 to 2009–2010

	2003–2004	2004–2005	2005–2006	2006–2007	2007–2008	2008–2009	2009–2010
Looked after at home	741,289	8,695,588	1,148,114	1,289,172	1,390,947	1,637,344	1,885,995
	875,506	1,039,386	1,353,838	1,542,660	1,661,221	1,936,763	2,218,267
	(84.7)	(83.7)	(84.8)	(83.6)	(83.7)	(84.5)	(85.0)
Looked after away from home	845,810	951,771	1,043,879	1,202,820	1,364,676	1,461,395	1,536,720
	924,890	1,041,479	1,141,214	1,309,117	1,476,097	1,577,962	1,653,238
	(91.4)	(91.4)	(91.5)	(91.9)	(92.5)	(92.6)	(93.0)
Not looked after	237,720,960	238,988,487	2,362,224,933	234,687,637	232,233,204	228,462,656	224,270,740
	25,400,801	257,053,207	253,714,954	251,542,618	248,892,603	244,551,180	240,310,012
	(93.1)	(93.0)	(93.1)	(93.3)	(93.3)	(93.4)	(93.3)

Note: Figures show actual half days' attendance, possible half days' attendance and percentage attendance (in brackets).

Table 2.   Exclusions from School of Looked-after and Non-looked-after Children, 2003–2004 to 2008–2009. These are Instances of Exclusion and Include Repeated Exclusion of the Same Students.

	2002–2003	2003–2004	2004–2005	2005–2006	2006–2007	2007–2008	2008–2009
Number of exclusions	1819	1396	2601	3046	3787	3938	3853
Rate looked after 'at home'	–	242	325	333	358	522	433
Rate looked after 'away from home'	–	264	354	341	380	359	325
Rate non-looked-after	50	53	58	60	64	58	50

Rate: rate per thousand exclusions.
Source: www.scotland.gov.uk/Topics/Statistics/Browse/School-Education/PubExclusions

The rates of exclusion of both looked-after and non-looked-after children rose from 2003 to 2004 and peaked in 2006–2007. One explanation is that this is indicative of an increase in indiscipline in schools. Nevertheless, the fall in rates noted in the following two years parallels official intolerance of exclusion as a remedy for in-school behaviour problems. What is also obvious from the table is the significantly higher rate of exclusion of looked-after children. The method of calculating the rate of exclusion of looked-after children changed in 2007–2008, and the more recent statistics are regarded by government statisticians as being more accurate. For this reason, 2007–2008 will be the index year for future comparisons. The 2008–2009 figures show a substantial fall on the previous year, and although welcome it is too soon to know if this is the beginning of improvement. A second observation is that the exclusion rate for those looked after away from home was consistently and appreciably higher than for those in the at home category until 2007–2008, when the trend reversed. The most recent figures showing higher exclusion rates for children looked after at home are consistent with other poorer outcomes for this group. The change in the method of collection does not explain the apparently higher rates for those looked after away from home in the earlier statistics. One suggested explanation, which cannot be verified, is that schools may have been more inclined to exclude a looked-after pupil where a foster or residential carer was readily available. If this is a likely explanation, perhaps the practice is also now less likely to occur as a result of better briefing and exposure to training.

Attainment

A standard measure of attainment that has been reported annually is 'the academic attainment of young people aged 16 or over who ceased to be looked after during the year'. Table 3 shows a comparison of the percentages of care leavers on three metrics—those gaining no awards as a result of taking external examinations administered by the Scottish Qualifications' Agency,[6] those who gained at least one

Table 3.   Academic Attainment of Care Leavers Over 16 in Scotland: Change from 2002–2003 to 2007–2008

	2002–2003[a]		2005–2006		2007–2008	
	Home	Away	Home	Away	Home	Away
No awards	67%	47%	386 (55%)	242 (43%)	389 (55%)	223 (39%)
At least one award at Level 3 or higher	33%	53%	319 (45%)	320 (57%)	322 (45%)	353 (61%)
English and Math at Level 3 or higher[b]	27%		195 (28%)	231 (41%)	182 (26%)	263 (46%)

[a]The total number of care leavers in 2002–2003 was 1138. Only percentages were presented within categories in the statistical report. The proportion gaining both English and Maths was not reported by home and away from home.
[b]Level 3 qualifications are equivalent to General Certificate of Secondary Education (GCSE) qualifications in the other countries of the UK.

award at the most basic level (known as Scottish Credit and Qualification Framework [SCQF] Level 3[7]) or higher, and those gaining awards in both English and mathematics at the most basic level or higher—in 2003, 2006 and 2008 (Scottish Executive, 2003, 2006; Scottish Government, 2010a). The most striking feature of this table is the high proportion of care leavers who gained no qualifications by the time they left school compared with 3.3% of all children in Scotland who left school in 2008 without qualifications (Scottish Government, 2010d). Also evident is the significantly lower attainment of young people looked after away from home, compared with those placed in out of home care. Nevertheless, the table shows encouraging signs of non-trivial improvement in attainment during this relatively short five-year period.

Conclusion

The low attainment of looked-after children in Scotland persists and, therefore, it remains an important cause for public concern and an embarrassing indicator of social injustice in a country which is traditionally proud of its strong commitment to education and the rights of children. The low attainment is reflected in the small proportion of looked-after children progressing directly from school to higher education—around 3% of all looked-after children, compared with 36% of non-looked-after children—and the high proportion who are neither in education nor in employment upon leaving school—36% compared with 11% of non-looked-after children (Scottish Government, 2009b).

There is evidence in official statistics to show that in relation to attendance and attainment the trend in Scotland is beginning to move in the right direction, even if the gap between looked-after children and their non-looked-after peers is still unacceptably large. This change is also consistent with improvements noted in

England (Brodie, 2010). In Scotland, children living in out of home care, looked after by residential, foster and kinship carers, now have school attendance which is as good as that achieved by children who are not looked after. Almost half of this sub-set of looked-after children now leaves school with a qualification in both mathematics and English, the proportion having increased from 41 to 46% of the cohort in just two years. The careers agency, Skills Development Scotland, has not so far distinguished between the categories looked after at home and away from home in its reports of destination surveys; if it did these would undoubtedly show improvements in entry to further and higher education from the out of home care group. These findings provide evidence of the advantages conferred by out of home care; for example, Forrester *et al.*, in a review of 12 studies in England and Wales, concluded that while children who entered public care tended to have serious problems, their welfare typically improved over time (Forrester *et al.*, 2009). It is important that this message is understood by politicians and practitioners who would argue for a reduction in the use of out of home care for financial or ideological reasons.

It is also clear that significantly more effort should be made to understand the particular support needs in education of children looked after while remaining in the family home and this aspect needs to be given substantially greater attention by researchers so that there is a secure basis for developing practice. This observation also raises important questions, answers to which should inform a debate about the consequences, particularly in terms of educational attainment, of maintaining children at home in circumstances which are stressful and chaotic.

Children become looked after because of neglect and trauma and the developmental effects of such assaults on childhood, combined with disrupted school attendance, inevitably affect progress in education and eventual attainment. As this paper has shown, there has been considerable investment in the past decade in Scotland in developing the policy and practice infrastructure needed to support improvement. There is evidence of improvement in outcomes. What is not well understood is how the policy changes have impacted on organisational change and developments in practice. Better understanding is needed to ensure that the improvement trajectory is both maintained and accelerated.

Notes

[1]   The framework for school improvement in Scotland is known by the general name, How Good is our School? For more information see: www.hmie.gov.uk/Generic/HGIOS

[2]   See: www.sircc.org.uk/lacsig

[3]   'Bairn' is a Scots dialect word used, particularly in north and east Scotland, for 'child'.

[4]   A co-ordinated support plan is the highest level of intervention where 'significant' additional support needs are identified and where professional support from at least one other agency besides education is indicated. It has statutory backing.

[5]   See: www.nationalcarestandards.org/

[6]   See: www.sqa.org.uk/sqa/CCC_FirstPage.jsp

[7]   For information about the Scottish Credit and Qualifications Framework see: www.scqf.org.uk/

References

Bayes, K. (2009) *Higher Aspirations, Brighter Futures: National Residential Child Care Initiative Overview Report*, SIRCC, Glasgow.

Berridge, D. (1985) *Children's Homes*, Basil Blackwell, Oxford.

Berridge, D. & Brodie, I. (1998) *Children's Homes Revisited*, Jessica Kingsley, London.

Borland, M., Pearson, C., Hill, M. & Bloomfield, I. (1998) *Education and Care Away from Home: A Review of Policy, Practice and Research*, Scottish Council for Research in Education, Edinburgh.

Boyce, P. (2004) *A Different Class? Educational Attainment: The Views and Experiences of Looked After Young People*, Who Cares? Scotland, Glasgow.

Brodie, I. (2010) *Improving Educational Outcomes for Looked After Children and Young People*, Services, C.F.E.a.O.I.C.a.Y.P.S, London.

Centre for Excellence and Outcomes in Children's Services. (2008) *Narrowing the Gap*, Services, C.F.E.a.O.I.C.S, London.

Connelly, G. (2003) 'Developing quality indicators for learning with care', *Scottish Journal of Residential Child Care*, vol. 2, no. 2, pp. 69–78.

Connelly, G., Forrest, J., Furnivall, J., Siebelt, L., Smith, I. & Seagraves, L. (2008) *The Educational Attainment of Looked After Children Local Authority Pilot Projects: Final Research Report*, The Scottish Government, Edinburgh.

Connelly, G., McKay, E. & O'Hagan, P. (2003) *Learning With Care: Information for Carers, Social Workers and Teachers Concerning the Education of Looked After Children And Young People*, University of Strathclyde, Glasgow.

Department of Education and Skills. (2007) 'Care matters: time for change', in *Skills*, ed. D.O.E.A., Department of Education and Skills, London.

Department of Health Social Services and Public Safety Northern Ireland. (2007) *Care Matters in Northern Ireland: A Bridge to a Better Future*, Northern Ireland Assembly, Belfast.

Duncalf, Z. (2010) *Listen up! Adult Care Leavers Speak Out: The Views of 310 Care Leavers Aged 17–78*, Care Leavers' Association, Manchester.

European Commission. (2008) *Child Poverty and Well-being in the EU: Current Status and Way Forward*, European Commission, Luxembourg.

European Commission. (2009) *Eurobarometer Survey on Poverty and Social Exclusion*, Publications Office of the European Union, Luxembourg.

Forrester, D., Goodman, K., Cocker, C., Binnie, C. & Jensch, G. (2009) 'What is the impact of public care on children's welfare? A review of research findings from England and Wales and their policy implications', *Journal of Social Policy*, vol. 38, no. 3, pp. 439–456.

Francis, J. (2008) 'Developing inclusive education policy and practice for looked after children', *Scottish, Journal of Residential Child Care*, vol. 7, no. 1, pp. 60–70.

Francis, J., Thomson, G. O. B. & Mills, S. (1996) *The Quality of the Educational Experience of Children in Care*, University of Edinburgh, Edinburgh.

Furnivall, J., Connelly, G., Hudson, B. & McCann, G. (2008) *Looked After Children and Young People: We Can and Must Do Better Training Materials DVD-ROM*, The Scottish Government, Edinburgh.

Furnivall, J. & Hudson, B. (2003) 'The learning with care training materials', *Scottish Journal of Residential Child Care*, vol. 2, no. 2, pp. 63–68.

Gallagher, B., Brannan, C., Jones, R. & Westwood, S. (2004) 'Good practice in the education of children in residential care', *British Journal of Social Work*, vol. 34, no. 8, pp. 1133–1160.

Gudbrandson, B. (2007) *Rights of Children at Risk and in Care*, Council of Europe Publishing, Paris.

Guthrie, T. (2011) *Social Work Law in Scotland*, 3rd edn, Haywards Heath, Bloomsbury.

Happer, H., McCreadie, J. & Aldgate, J. (2006) *Celebrating Success: What Helps Looked After Children Succeed*. Social Work Inspection Agency, Edinburgh.

Her Majesty's Inspectorate of Education. (2008) *Count Us In: Improving the Education of Our Looked After Children*, HMIE, Edinburgh.

Her Majesty's Inspectorate of Education. (2009) *Improving Services for Children: How Good is our Corporate Parenting?* HMIE, Edinburgh.

Her Majesty's Inspectorate of Education. (2010) *Review of the Additional Support for Learning Act: Adding Benefits for Learners.* HMIE, Edinburgh.

Her Majesty's Inspectorate of Schools. (2003) *Inclusion and Equality. Part 1: Evaluating Education and Care Placements for Looked After Children and Young People.* HMIE, Edinburgh.

Her Majesty's Inspectors of Schools and Social Work Services Inspectorate. (2001) *Learning with Care: The Education of Children Looked After Away from Home by Local Authorities*, HMI and SWSI, Edinburgh.

Hoskins, B. (2008) 'The discourse of social justice within European education policy developments: the example of key competences and indicator development towards assuring the continuation of democracy', *European Educational Research Journal*, vol. 7, no. 3, pp. 319–330.

Jacklin, A., Robinson, C. & Torrance, H. (2006) 'When lack of data is data: do we really know who our looked-after children are?', *European Journal of Special Needs Education*, vol. 21, no. 1, pp. 1–20.

Jackson, S. (1987) *The Education of Children in Care*, School of Applied Social Studies, University of Bristol, Bristol.

Jackson, S. & Martin, P. Y. (1998) 'Surviving the care system: education and resilience', *Journal of Adolescence*, vol. 21, pp. 569–583.

Jackson, S. & McParlin, P. (2006) 'The education of children in care', *The Psychologist*, vol. 19, no. 2, pp. 90–93.

Kahan, B. (1994) *Growing Up in Groups*, HMSO, London.

Maclean, K. & Gunion, M. (2003) 'Learning with care: the education of children looked after away from home by local authorities', *Adoption & Fostering*, vol. 27, no. 2, pp. 20–31.

Ritchie, A. (2003) *Care to Learn? The Educational Experiences of Children and Young People Who are Looked After*, S.T.C.a.W.C, Edinburgh.

Roby, D. E. (2004) 'Research on school attendance and student achievement: a study of Ohio schools', *Educational Research Quarterly*, vol. 28, no. 1, pp. 3–16.

Scottish Executive. (1999) *Social Justice: A Scotland Where Everyone Matters*, The Scottish Executive, Edinburgh.

Scottish Executive. (2001) Special schoolbooks fund for kids in care: news release se4195/2001, [Online] Available at: http://www.scotland.gov.uk/pages/news/2001/10/SE4195.aspx.

Scottish Executive. (2003) *Children's Social Work Statistics 2002–03*, The Scottish Executive, Edinburgh.

Scottish Executive. (2006) *Children Looked After 2005–06*, The Scottish Executive, Edinburgh.

Scottish Executive. (2007) *Looked After Children & Young People: We Can and Must Do Better*, The Scottish Executive, Edinburgh.

Scottish Government. (2008a) *Core Tasks for Designated Managers in Educational and Residential Establishments in Scotland*, The Scottish Government, Edinburgh.

Scottish Government. (2008b) *Looked After Children and Young People: Working Together to Improve Outcomes*, The Scottish Government, Edinburgh.

Scottish Government. (2008c) *These are Our Bairns: A Guide for Community Planning Partnerships on Being a Good Corporate Parent*, The Scottish Government, Edinburgh.

Scottish Government. (2009a) *Attendance and Absence in Scottish Schools 2008/09*, The Scottish Government, Edinburgh.

Scottish Government. (2009b) *Destinations of Leavers from Scottish Schools 2008/09*, The Scottish Government, Edinburgh.

Scottish Government. (2009c) *The Educational Outcomes of Scotland's Looked After Children and Young People: A New Reporting Framework*, The Scottish Government, Edinburgh.

Scottish Government. (2010a) *Children Looked After Statistics 2008–09*, The Scottish Government, Edinburgh.

Scottish Government. (2010b) *Code of Practice: Supporting Children's Learning: Statutory Guidance Relating to the Education (Additional Support for Learning) (Scotland) Act 2004 as Amended*, The Scottish Government, Edinburgh.

Scottish Government. (2010c) *Exclusions from Schools 2008/09*, The Scottish Government, Edinburgh.

Scottish Government. (2010d) *SQA Attainment and School Leaver Qualifications in Scotland 2008/ 09*, The Scottish Government, Edinburgh.

Scottish Government. (2011a) *Children Looked After Statistics 2009–10*, The Scottish Government, Edinburgh.

Scottish Government. (2011b) *Included, Engaged and Involved: A Positive Approach to Managing School Exclusions*, The Scottish Government, Edinburgh.

Scottish Government. (2011c) *The Vital Importance of Getting It Right for Every Child and Young Person*, The Scottish Government, Edinburgh.

Scottish Parliament Public Audit Committee. (2011) *Getting it Right for Children in Residential Care: SP Paper 586*, The Scottish Parliament, Edinburgh.

UN General Assembly. (1989) *Convention on the Rights of the Child*, OHCHR, Geneva.

Vincent, S. (2004) *Looking After Children in Scotland: Good Parenting, Good Outcomes: Report on File Audit of Local Authorities' Use of Looking After Children Materials*. The Scottish Executive, Edinburgh.

Welsh Assembly Government. (2007) *Towards a Stable Life and a Brighter Future*, Welsh Assembly Government, Cardiff.

The managerialist turn and the education of young offenders in state care

A inflexão gerencialista e a educação de menores delinquentes sob custódia do Estado

Tiago Neves

Managerialism has become a major trait of youth justice systems throughout Europe over the past couple of decades. This has taken place in the wider context of significant changes in criminal justice systems, which in their turn are articulated with the rise of neo-liberalism. There has been a shift from a humanistic penal welfarism strongly predicated on state interventions, and aimed at the social reintegration of offenders, to a containment regime focused mostly on social control, risk management and the reduction of insecurity. Based on ethnographic work carried out in a detention and education centre for juvenile offenders in Portugal, this paper presents and discusses the ways in which this managerialist turn impacts on the education of youths in custodial state care. Specifically, it focuses on the downgrading of educational expectations, the relegation of schooling to a matter of low priority, and the decline of the rehabilitation ideal. The implications of this managerialist turn for professional practice are also discussed.

Nas últimas décadas, o managerialismo tornou-se um traço central dos sistemas de justiça juvenil europeus. Isto aconteceu no quadro mais alargado de transformações significativas nos sistemas de justiça criminal, que por sua vez se articulam com a escalada do neo-liberalismo. Verificou-se uma passagem de uma abordagem penal humanista, fortemente ancorada em intervenções estatais e dirigida à reinserção social dos ofensores, para um regime de contenção focado essencialmente no controlo social, na gestão do risco e na redução da insegurança. Com base em trabalho etnográfico conduzido num Centro Educativo em Portugal, este artigo apresenta e discute os modos através dos quais esta inflexão managerialista se repercute na educação dos jovens sob custódia do Estado. Especificamente, o artigo analisa a diminuição das expectativas educacionais, a relegação da escola e o declínio do ideal da reabilitação. São igualmente debatidas as implicações desta inflexão managerialista para a prática profissional.

Introduction

Managerialism has become a major trait of youth justice systems throughout Europe over the past couple of decades (Fox, 2005; Muncie, 2006; Muncie & Goldson, 2006; Bailleau & Cartuyvels, 2007; Bailleau *et al.*, 2009; Castro, 2009). This has happened in the wider context of significant shifts in criminal justice systems, which in their turn are articulated with the rise of neo-liberalism (Feeley & Simon, 1992; Wacquant, 2000; Garland, 2001). In brief, this has meant a shift from a humanistic penal welfarism firmly grounded in state interventions, and aimed at the social reintegration of offenders, to a containment regime focused mostly on social control, risk management and the reduction of insecurity (Garland, 2001). According to Wacquant (2001), this echoes the move from a Keynesian to a Darwinian state, that is, from a state based on solidarity and aiming at reduction of inequalities to a 'state that makes a fetish of competition and celebrates individual responsibility (whose counterpart is collective irresponsibility), and which withdraws into its kingly functions of "law and order"' (Wacquant, 2001, p. 405).

This paper argues that this managerialist approach has important consequences for the education of institutionalised youths. The difficulties for children and youth in care to achieve educational success are not new and have been documented (Martin & Jackson, 2002; Berridge, 2007; Jackson, 2010). It is also true that such difficulties loom even larger in secure juvenile facilities where, due to their own nature, safety and security issues often supplant educational concerns (Stein & Dixon, 2006; Neves, 2008; Houchins *et al.*, 2009; Mathur & Schoenfeld, 2010). Furthermore, as discussed below, rates of educational failure correlate positively with entrance into the juvenile justice system (INE, 2009). This means that, at the moment of institutionalisation, the educational qualifications of these youths are usually already below average, and thus low qualifications seem to emerge as a precipitating factor in criminalisation.

However, given that the decline of the rehabilitation ideal and the rise of managerialism brought about a renewed, stronger legitimacy for securitarian concerns (Fox, 2005; Muncie, 2006; Bradt & Bouverne-De Bie, 2009; Rogowski, 2010), both schooling and intervention in the specific needs of young offenders through training (and/or treatment) can be more easily sidelined.

This paper also makes reference to consequences of the managerialist turn for professional practice. To be sure, besides youth and adult justice, managerialism has invaded other core fields of social work, namely child protection (Littlechild, 2008). Professionals are now increasingly absorbed by managerial and administrative tasks aimed at the bureaucratic preservation of organisations and systems, rather than by direct work with children and youths. Singh and Cowden (2009) go as far as to speak of the 'de-intellectualisation of social work' entailed in the current dominance of the managerial language of 'performance', 'targets' and 'customer service'. This process removes social justice and social change from centre stage. It is no wonder, then, that the implications of this managerialist turn for the social work profession have deserved critical attention (Lorenz, 2005; Field, 2007; Bradt & Bouverne-De Bie, 2009; Brookfield, 2009).

The role ascribed to education and rehabilitation in detention facilities is surely one of the classical dilemmas in the history of modern justice and punishment systems[1] (Foucault, 1997; Garland, 2001). Certainly, managerialism is not the source of this dilemma. In fact, it even offers a kind of answer for it. To use managerialist language, the 'core-business' of detention facilities is identified as the provision of safety and security to 'customers'. Elements that are not a part of the 'core-business' and, furthermore, are hard to tackle are seen as unworthy of relevant 'investment'. The managerialist answer, then, consists basically of glossing over the dilemma. Based on ethnographic work carried out in a detention and education centre (DEC) for juvenile offenders, this paper explores and critically analyses what happens while this dilemma is downplayed daily. After a brief presentation of the research method and context, the paper deals first with the implications of the managerialist turn for the redefinition of the workings and goals of these DECs, and juvenile justice in general. It then analyses how the managerialist turn impacts on educational issues. It concludes with a brief analysis of the consequences of managerialism for professional practice.

Context and Method

Participant observation and the 'thick description' it enables are the heart of ethnography (Hammersley & Atkinson, 1983; Van Maanen, 1988; Geertz, 1993). In simple words, yet eloquently, Willis and Trondman (2000, pp. 5–12) state what ethnography is about:

> Most importantly it is a family of methods involving direct and sustained social contact with agents, and of richly writing up the encounter, respecting, recording, representing at least partly in its own terms, the irreducibility of human

experience. (...) Most basically we are interested in recording and presenting the 'nitty gritty' of everyday life, of how 'the meat is cut close to the bone' in ordinary cultural practices, and presenting them in ways which produce maximum 'illumination' for readers.

A reflexive ethnography sees the ethnographer as part and parcel of the research context, and understands that the research product cannot be detached from the research process (Hammersley & Atkinson, 1983; Bourdieu, 2001). Reflexive, critical ethnography posits the ideological nature, the situated character and the bounded rationality of knowledge about the world. It does not take the world, or our representations of it, as a natural given. It systematically asks how things come to be. As a result, it is very much interested in power issues, including those posed by the ethnographic method itself (Kincheloe & McLaren, 1998). To be sure, ethnography has been unable to provide perfect solutions for the problems of cultural translation or ethnographic obtrusiveness and manipulation, among others (Fine, 1993). However, as a way of making sense of the world, ethnography stands at the antipodes of the disingenuous, normalising and one-dimensional managerialist discourse and gaze (Brookfield, 2009; Singh & Cowden, 2009). In this specific piece of research, as part of the process of addressing some of the difficulties mentioned above, the final report was discussed with the Director of the DEC and, throughout the research period, fieldnotes were shown to and discussed with some of the institutionalised youngsters.

Over a period of 10 months, the author conducted ethnographic research in a DEC for youth offenders. This kind of centre fits with Goffman's definition of 'total institutions' as 'a place of residence and work where a large number of like-situated individuals, cut-off from the wider society for an appreciable period of time, together lead an enclosed, formally administered round of life' (1971, p. 11).

After being given formal permission by the Ministry of Justice to contact the DEC for research purposes, meetings were held with the board of the DEC to discuss the manner in which the study could be carried out. Staff were duly informed of the research and introductory meetings were arranged with the youths in order to explain the research purposes and plan, and most crucially to gain their consent to the ethnographer's presence in their living quarters.[2] No objections were raised. In retrospect, the author came to understand that the presence of someone who belonged to neither group was actually regarded as a source of fresh air both for staff and inmates, locked as they are into the dyadic and unequal relationship typical of total institutions (Goffman, 1971). The ethnographer's status was thus completely overt to all members of staff and to the youths, and access was gained by making it very clear from the start of the research who the author was and what he was doing there.

The researcher was given *carte blanche* by the board of the DEC: that is, the researcher could enter and leave the DEC at any time and also move around freely, providing, of course, his presence was accepted by the participants in a given situation. Participant observations were carried out in a variety of settings from

7:30 am to 22 pm, on weekdays and weekends. The researcher attended school and professional training classes in a variety of subjects, had meals together with the youths, watched television, listened to music, played a variety of sports (football, table-tennis, billiards…), attended parties (Christmas, Halloween…), spent time chatting with the youngsters, staff and teachers and also spent time doing nothing—a very ethnographic thing to do. The average length of daily stays in the field was 5 hours.

An effort was made to demonstrate that the ethnographer's relational and moral values were not necessarily those enforced by institutional staff nor those followed by the youths. For example, although smoking tobacco was not allowed, the researcher made it clear to the youths that he would not tell the staff if he saw them smoking; he would tell, however, if they got involved in serious fighting. This gained the ethnographer the respect from those with less power—that is, the inmate youths— and an occasional temporary fall out with a given member of staff, who in one situation found the ethnographer not to be disclosing all the information he had access to.

The DEC where the research was carried out had capacity for 34 male juveniles. The occupation rate throughout the research period was approximately 90%. The average age of the juveniles was 15.7 years and more than half of them were 15 or 16 years old. Regarding the main reasons for custody, 70% were detained for crimes against property, 12% for assault and another 12% for drug-related matters. The average detention period was 16 months. With regard to their ethnic origin, 65% of the youths were Caucasian, 29% black and 6% gypsies. There was, then, a huge over-representation of black and gypsies youth in proportion to the overall Portuguese population.

The Managerialist Turn: From Welfare to Risk Management

It was the 2001 reform of the Portuguese juvenile system that, in line with changes that had been taking place elsewhere in Europe (Bailleau & Cartuyvels, 2007), turned DECs into 'total institutions' similar to adult prisons. Before that, welfare was the dominant model. Both children at risk and youth offenders were regarded as victims of society (Bradt & Bouverne-De Bie, 2009). By and large, they were subject to the same laws, provided with the same education and offered the same residential care. Educational and residential measures involved detailed analysis of the personality and living conditions of the youths (Bailleau & Cartuyvels, 2007). The welfare goals were protection, prevention, rehabilitation. Officially at least, deprivation of freedom was to be avoided.

In the welfare model, however, educational and residential measures were of indeterminate length, and fundamental legal rights such as the 'audi alteram partem' (the right to a fair hearing, giving all parties the opportunity to respond to the evidence against them) were commonly overlooked. Also, due process was abandoned in favour of an informal approach. In a rudimentary regime of corporatist welfare such as Portugal, where the lines between the formal, professional and informal care are traditionally blurred, this informality was even more apparent (Meeuwisse & Swärd, 2007). Increasingly, the welfare model in youth justice became subject to criticism. From the left there were accusations of professionals informally extending the social control of the State; the right claimed the model was soft, paternalistic and ineffective in curbing delinquency (Muncie & Goldson, 2006). Gradually, as welfare values waned, a 'culture of control' settled in (Garland, 2001).

This 'culture of control' is characterised by an increase in managerial procedures and securitarian concerns. Such concerns are dealt with through an increasingly harsh punishment and a sophistication of risk management. This is reflected in a number of ways in the field of youth justice. To begin with, young offenders are now seen as risks to society (Bradt & Bouverne-De Bie, 2009), as social problems (Bailleau et al., 2009). Simultaneously, as collective responsibility crumbles, youths are held individually responsible for their behaviour. The activation principle, which is now common in social policies and involves a demand for increased individual responsibility in gaining access to work and social participation, is also present in the field of youth justice (Bailleau et al., 2009). In the words of a member of the board of the DEC:

> First of all, the purpose of the DEC is to isolate [the youths] from society, to protect society from what they might be doing if they were outside. Reintegration is then something that depends on the structure, on the personality of each one of them.

Rather than the future rehabilitation of youth offenders, the goal is now the maximisation of security (Fox, 2005). Residential care turns into secure accommodation (Francis et al., 2007). A number of features of the DEC where the research was conducted coincide to make it an intensely 'defensible space' (Brantingham & Brantingham, 1981): high walls and fences, unbreakable windows, metal bars on every window, gated corridors, locked doors, individual cells, concrete beds, stainless steel toilet sinks, reflective metal sheets instead of glass mirrors, plastic cutlery and security staff. Inmates must be under close visual supervision of the staff at all times, and time is meticulously organised into a set of continuous activities with compulsory participation. At night, each youngster is locked in his own private cell.

At the same time, however, it is true the managerialist turn has brought about increased respect for due process and children's rights. This is apparent in a number of aspects: youngsters are now entitled to legal representation, they are judged in court, and sentences have a definite length. Beforehand, in Portugal, sentences were produced without a proper trial in a court of law, no evidence of the offence had to be produced, and release from custody was dependent on evaluation by the institution. It must also be made clear that the securitarian features mentioned above do not reflect a cruel model that takes pleasure in punishing offenders, or even a purely 'just deserts' retributive justice model (Muncie, 2006; Rogowski, 2010).

It is worth mentioning that when the author set out to undertake this piece of research, his ambition was to describe and analyse the educational model at work in the DEC, which he had hypothesised to be the organising principle of life in the institution. Actually, however, no clear educational model was found, which in itself is a sign of the downgrading of the educational realm. Instead, serving above all the goal of preserving the stability of the DEC's ecosystem, it was the securitarian features that were found to be integral to the fundamental drive of the DEC: 'institutional defence' (Neves, 2008). Institutional defence refers to the process whereby detention facilities concentrate most of their efforts in safeguarding themselves against the risks, the potential threats that are taken to be lurking inside them. This seems to be a minimalist, disenchanted, selfish goal. At the same time, it is also a managerialist goal. It sets quantifiable targets on easily collectable data, such as violent incidents and escape attempts. It depicts operations based on input and output figures that seldom describe what is really going on. It standardises practices, thereby curbing the autonomy of professionals, sharpening their accountability and reinforcing hierarchies (Raine & Willson, 1996). It centralises decision-making and cuts costs; in Portugal, the number of DECs has been cut by 40% over the past decade, and a couple of them have been allocated to private management. It focuses mostly on short-term, internally controllable objectives and disregards events and consequences that take place beyond immediate responsibility to 'consumers', whether they are the youngsters or society at large. The absence of data on recidivism is a sign of just that.

As Muncie and Hughes argue, the key concern of managerialism 'is maintaining internal system coherence' (2004, p. 5). It presents itself as an 'objective, technically neutral mechanism, dedicated only to greater efficiency; the one best method' (Ball, 1990, p. 157). This seems naive, at best. Critical reflection on both the concept and its consequences (Askeland & Fook, 2009) elicits questions like: what works for whom? Whose best interest is protected? Is it the youngsters'? Is it the staff's? Is it society's best interest? Or is it the interest of the hierarchy above the DEC?

The result of the merger between the securitarian concerns of the culture of control and managerialist pragmatism is a disenchanted and rather hopeless belief that the best that can be done is to manage deviant groups and their associated risks. To be sure, there are tensions and contradictions within the managerialist culture of control. Increased punitiveness is offset by greater adherence to due legal processes and international children's rights conventions (Muncie & Goldson, 2006). Also, retributive justice features are counterbalanced by the rise of restorative justice (Muncie, 2006; Littlechild, 2009). In Portugal, the tension is also between the nostalgia for a formal welfare system that was never really implemented and the lack of power-knowledge conditions to put into practice the most progressive features of today's juvenile justice law (Santos, 1999; Castro, 2009). Indeed, of all the educational and training programmes for institutionalised youths defined by the 2001 law, which is applicable to minors who commit offences between the ages of 12 and 16 years, those that are meant to address the specific needs of young offenders are not carried out in the DECs. That is, youths do attend school and professional training, practice sports and learn arts, but do not attend programmes on topics such as victims' interests, conflict resolution, anger management, social values or legal norms.

The Implications of the Managerialist Turn for Education

Typically, 'education' refers to a number of different things in detention facilities for young people. It refers to schooling, to be sure, but also to some kinds of resocialisation schemes. Professional training (not addressed in this paper) is also a frequent educational feature in this kind of facility. Resocialisation has generally been regarded as the distinctive educational aspect of the youth justice system (Cusson, 1974). However, resocialisation efforts are prey to a structural paradox: the goal of developing the youngsters' autonomous ethical behaviour clashes with them being stripped of nearly all autonomy in the daily life of 'total institutions' (Cusson, 1974). As Halsey and Armitage argue, there is an 'uncomfortable juxtaposition of incapacitation (degradation of self) and reformation (recovery of self in connection with care from other)' (2009, p. 169).

Managerialism, however, sits quite comfortably within this paradox. It does so by downgrading educational expectations. In the DEC where the research was conducted, efforts aimed at deeper rehabilitation are replaced by law-related education. That is, rather than aiming at the internalisation of ethical principles, the goal is simply to promote the external, behavioural observance of legal interdicts (Neves, 2008). Managerialist pragmatism is strikingly evident here. An omnipresent dichotomy between what is allowed and what is forbidden to youngsters is a crucial element of the organisation of the DEC's daily life. That, together with the stripping of autonomy, the degradation of the self and the constant surveillance, leads to a feeling of unbearableness that has educational consequences:

> [chatting with a juvenile] When I try to understand his view on the purpose of detention at the DEC, he replies quickly: 'Being here is pointless'. He sits silent for a moment, and then proceeds, reformulating his idea: 'We are here to learn that we did something wrong and to improve'. And then he adds: 'But we can't keep thinking about why we're here, or we'll just crack up . . . We must forget why we're here'.

Also, the behavioural observance of legal interdicts sometimes amounts to a mere instrumental facade. In fact, law-related education anchored in risk management hardly engenders more than risk evaluation by the youths:

> This 'partner' Chico talks about has already promised him 400 euro so that he can get on with his business when he leaves the DEC. Chico tells me he wants to invest that money in drugs to begin regaining his old clients (. . .). And Chico adds: 'Because when I get out I'll have a clean sheet [criminal record], if I get caught again in principle they'll let me go and won't send me to [adult] prison . . .

It must be stressed that there is no pedagogical programme or evaluation method for law-related education. It takes place in an informal, unstructured and sparse fashion. In its implementation, it does not differ from another aspect of the emphasis on external adaptation to context: the way the DEC resembles a 'finishing school' (Goffman, 1971, p. 45).

'Leonel pulls a pillow down to the floor, by the couch. He plans to lie down on the floor. Elisa, the monitor, tells him he is not allowed to do that. He puts the pillow back in its place, without protesting. (. . .) Elisa later tells me it is necessary to have firm rules and never break them, because 'if the kids we have here now are not particularly violent or aggressive, what happens if we get one of those?"

The continuous judgement of behaviour, dress and manners, just like the incessant demarcation of what is allowed and what is forbidden, both reinforces and is reinforced by two themes of life in secure care: the overt power imbalance between staff and inmates, and the infantilisation of residents (Halsey & Armitage, 2009). Also, the finishing school and the allowed/forbidden dichotomy mirror power relations more than meaningful relationships. Given the high rate of recurrence of conflicts, it would be relevant to try to transform those power relations into meaningful relationships. In this sense, Littlechild's (2009) suggestion of developing 'relational conflict resolution' in these settings appears quite reasonable. The author of this paper—himself a trained mediator—also made some attempts, with motivating results, at mediation in the DEC towards the end of the research period. Developing conflict resolution as an educational strategy, however, requires qualified staff. This is not achievable while the more qualified technical staff at the DEC— social workers and psychologists—are, for most of their time, allocated to managerial or administrative tasks. Monitors without any specific academic or professional training are the ones who really spend time with the youths. The monitors are well aware of this. One of them says:

They say this is an institution aimed at reintegration. I wish it was . . . We can only make do . . . .

In the same vein, another monitor argues that the good thing about work done at the DEC is:

(. . .) developing affective relationships with the youths, and the kids acknowl-edging when we're in a good or a bad day. Actual social reintegration, we don't do that. That would only be possible if we could work with them when they leave the DEC, but there are no resources for that . . .

These affective relationships, however crucial in this DEC, are much more casual and hazy than the therapeutic alliance between key staff members and youths described by Henriksen *et al.* (2008).

With regard to school education, its key role in social integration is widely acknowledged (Martin &Jackson, 2002; Vacca, 2008; Jackson, 2010). The fact that youths in secure accommodation, as well as in other forms of state care, have low achievement rates is a clear indication of that key role (Ball & Connolly, 2000; Mathur & Schoenfeld, 2010).

In Portugal, there were 157 youths attending school in DECs as of June 2007 (DGRS, 2008). The age distribution of those youths was the following: 2% were 12 or

13 years old, 33% were 14 or 15 years old, 48% were 16 or 17 years old and 17% were 18 or older (DGRS, 2008). This means that all the youths in DECs should have already finished primary school (first to fourth grade), and about 1% of them could still have been in the sixth grade. The reality, however, was very different: 13% attended primary school, 45% attended the fifth and sixth grades and the remaining 42% attended grades seven to nine. Also, global data on school attendance in Portugal show that, in 2007, only 2% of those who attended primary education were 12 years old, and only 12% of those who attended the fifth and sixth grades were 14 or older (INE, 2009). This is a clear substantiation of the aforementioned low achievement, and also of a positive correlation between rates of educational failure and entrance into the juvenile justice system. This positive correlation was also found in a previous study by Carvalho (2003). According to this author, in 2000 about 35% of the youths in custody were early school leavers and an impressive 69% had experienced retention (repeating a year) in school.

It is clear, then, that school-related difficulties of youth in custody are present before incarceration; rarely, however, do they get any considerable improvement during the custodial period. Some argue that children and youths who stay longer in care have better educational results than those who stay in care for shorter periods (Berridge, 2007). When it comes to custodial care for youths, however, it is difficult to believe that this would be the case. Moreover, extending its duration poses legal and ethical problems. Also, now that the youth justice model is essentially managerialist and more similar to the adult justice system, it is hard to imagine strictly educational, welfare measures being imposed on the youths after the end of their judicial sentences. In any case, in Portugal, at least, the current downgrading of educational expectations for youths in custody is so obvious that from 2008 onwards the official youth justice statistics stopped making reference to the school grade they attend.

In many ways, then, the school finds itself sidelined in the DEC. To begin with, although schools are usually regarded as the educational locations *par excellence*, the institutional assessment of the youths by the DEC is independent of how well they do in school. What matters is their behaviour, their adherence to institutional norms. Due to this, teachers and monitors are in a constant battle for the 'educator' status. Second, classrooms are like enclaves whose borders are constantly imploded by the surrounding environment:

> The class is interrupted twice by Elisabete, a monitor, once to tell something to the teacher and a second time to summon Mário for a consultation. Miguel, a resident, also enters the classroom twice, once for no apparent reason and again to pick up the English teacher's umbrella; that time he said 'Excuse me' as he entered the room. At a given point, André left the classroom saying he was going to the toilet; the teacher told him he was not allowed to leave but he left anyway, saying he'd be back. He eventually returned.

Third, there is no space or time for study outside scheduled classes. If a resident wishes to study, he must request either to be locked up in his room or for a classroom to be opened for him. Given the need for constant surveillance, such a request is unlikely to be granted.

In addition to these organisational features, there are difficulties stemming from the behaviour of the youths. They tend to concentrate for brief periods only, and their attention to teachers is intermittent at best.

> The class goes on in the usual fashion: students chatting loudly, throwing papers and other stuff to the dustbin, slapping the necks of the ones who are sitting in front of them . . . .

Also, the student–teacher relationship is characterised by recurring sexual insinuations. Adolescent boys holding a macho view of the world find in young female teachers an adequate target for their bravado:

> [the youths constantly try to find ways to tease the teacher]. For example, one asks what perfume she wears and how much does it cost. She replies she doesn't know the price, so they ask her if it was her husband who gave it to her. She says no, so they imply it was a lover. Another boy tells her she looks really good in the trousers she's wearing. Whenever she moves around the classroom, the boys all stare and make gestures of a sexual nature. When the teacher writes on the blackboard and turns her back to the students, Laranjinha grabs his desk and, lifting it with his legs, simulates sexual intercourse shouting 'Oh baby, yeah, yeah!' [in English].

The gender relegation of teachers thus adds to the institutional relegation of the school. Teachers find the whole situation hard to tackle. In an internal report, DEC teachers state that 'Generally speaking, these students lack minimal competencies in the several curricular courses (. . .). They are highly unmotivated, uncooperative, and sometimes aggressive and provocative'.

To be sure, neither the macho culture of the resident boys nor the old roots of their dissociation from school matters are the responsibility of the managerialist approach prevalent in DECs. Its responsibility lies instead with ignoring research on the characteristics of effective instruction (Martin & Jackson, 2002; Neves, 2008; Mathur & Schoenfeld, 2010), in being generally unsupportive of teachers, and in relegating academic issues, thus promoting the reproduction of low achievement in school.

The Implications of the Managerialist Turn for Professional Practice

If the relation between care and control is central to social work (Burford & Adams, 2004), the managerialist turn tips the balance in favour of control. As a result, and in line with the institutional defence process discussed earlier, professionals are led to making defensible rather than 'right' or risky decisions (Littlechild, 2008). In the case of the Portuguese DECs, this is further amplified by the vulnerability of staff to severe disciplinary measures. In a context where social work is intrumentalised for judicial aims, its 'emancipatory capacity' is on the line (Bradt & Bouverne-De Bie, 2009).

As the awareness of the social dimension of lives and relationships erodes in a background of rising individualism and individual responsibility, so does social work's ability to introduce change in the world (Lorenz, 2005). In fact, it is the 'social' dimension of 'work' that withers. More than holistic, applied social thinking, what is expected from care workers is individual case management. As a result, there is a scientific and professional demotion of social workers: anyone can do the job (Askeland & Fook, 2009). Actually, however, it could be argued that the current endorsement of individual responsibility is quite frail, even inconsequential: indeed, if not framed by collective hopes and goals, individual responsibility is quite sterile.

In the case of the DEC, imagining collective hopes and goals could be done at least at two different levels. At a macro level, related to the future of the youths and their role in society at large; at a micro level, referring to daily life inside the DEC. There would certainly be obstacles in putting such plans into practice, but just being able to consider them in disenchanted times such as these would be a triumph.

The professional practice of social workers—just like that of other professionals working in the 'social' dimension—requires a renewed sense of the power dynamics and relationships (Brookfield, 2009). As such, it is difficult to see how the status and the relevance of social workers can be maintained or enhanced unless critical, political reflection is embedded in their professional practice. In fact, what is at stake is not only the status and relevance of social workers, but the actual role of the public sector.

Conclusions

When Castel argued that the new social question consists in rationalising the presence of socially disqualified actors in the post-industrial society, in dissipating them through social policies aimed at activation and insertion, one could hint that a managerialist approach would be involved in the process (Castel, 2003, p. xxii). Social policies now pave the way for the production and application of differentiated, local criteria, based in reductionist definitions of 'what works'. In the case of the DEC, its educational timidity is augmented by the fact that its internal economy is largely severed from wider social networks. It is not the case that they do not exist or cannot be established; it is simply the case that they are irrelevant to satisfy the need for institutional defence. In many respects, the DEC is a world on its own. The 'social' dimension of work at the DEC erodes. In order to rescue this social dimension, one crucial area for improvement is preparing youths and their families for their return to life outside the DEC. 'What works' cannot be confined to the walls of the DEC and to micro-management procedures that, as professionals in different countries recognise, often lose sight of the youths themselves and generate professional frustration (Littlechild, 2008; Neves, 2008; Bradt & Bouverne-De Bie, 2009).

It is quite remarkable then, that as far as education in youth justice is concerned, the managerialist approach—often epitomised as 'the road to excellence' and the 'freedom to choose'—in reality amounts to a 'give less, demand less' strategy. Promoting changes in the lives of the incarcerated youths clearly involves more than establishing an adequate system of formal justice. It involves taking—and not simply containing—risks, and achieving a better balance between the judicial, the educational and the social dimensions.

Notes

[1]   Other classical dilemmas are, for example, the degree of visibility accorded to punishment practices and the definition of what constitutes proportionate retribution for a given offence.

[2]   In Portugal, Universities' Ethics Committees tend to play little or no role in the Social Sciences. The author recently had the opportunity of engaging in very interesting, and rather heated, debates on research ethics with colleagues from a UK University, where the situation is very different. Although the scope of such discussions extends well beyond the focus of this paper, two aspects deserve to be mentioned: ethics and morality are context-bound, and what is deemed ethical in Portugal, for example, might not be so in the UK and vice-versa; the strict adoption of what are currently deemed to be adequate ethics standards, as enforced by some Ethics Committees of the Saxon world, would have precluded the development of very relevant, unharmful ethnographic research on deviance (for example, Polsky 1971, Adler 1993, Bourgois 1996).

References

Adler, P. A. (1993) *Wheeling and Dealing – An Ethnography of an Upper Level Drug Dealing and Smuggling Community*, Columbia University Press, New York.

Askeland, G. & Fook, J. (2009) 'Editorial: critical reflection in social work', *European Journal of Social Work*, vol. 12, no. 3, pp. 287–292.

Bailleau, F., Cartuyvels, Y. & de Fraene, D. (2009) 'La criminalisation des mineurs et le jeu des sanctions [*The criminalisation of young offenders and the sanctions game*]', *Déviance et Société*, vol. 33, no. 3, pp. 255–269.

Bailleau, Y. & Cartuyvels, Y. (2007) 'La mise en question du modèle 'protectionnel' dans la justice des mineurs en Europe [*Challenging the 'protection' model in European youth justice*]', in *La justice pénale des mineurs en Europe: entre modèle welfare et inflexions néo-libérales* [*The penal justice of young offenders in Europe: Between the welfare model and the neo-liberal turn*], eds F. Bailleau & Y. Cartuyvels, L'Harmattan, Paris, pp. 7–19.

Ball, C. & Connolly, J. (2000) 'Educationally disaffected young offenders. Youth Court and agency responses to truancy and school exclusion', *British Journal of Criminology*, vol. 40, pp. 594–616.

Ball, S. J. (1990) 'Management as moral technology: a Luddite analysis', in *Foucault and Education: Disciplines and Knowledge*, ed. S. J. Ball, Routledge, London, pp. 153–166.

Berridge, D. (2007) 'Theory and explanation in child welfare: education and looked-after children', *Child and Family Social Work*, vol. 12, no. 1, pp. 1–10.

Bourdieu, P. (2001) *Science de la science et réflexivité* [*Science of science and reflexivity*], Raisons d'Agir Éditions, Paris.

Bourgois, P. (1996) *In Search of Respect – Selling Crack in El Barrio*, Cambridge University Press, Cambridge.

Bradt, L. & Bouverne-De Bie, M. (2009) 'Social work and the shift from 'welfare' to "justice"', *British Journal of Social Work*, vol. 39, no. 1, pp. 113–127.

Brantingham, P. J. & Brantingham, P. L. (1981) *Environmental Criminology*, Sage, London.

Brookfield, S. (2009) 'The concept of critical reflection: promises and contradictions', *European Journal of Social Work*, vol. 12, no. 3, pp. 293–304.

Burford, G. & Adams, P. (2004) 'Restorative justice, responsive regulation and social work', *Journal of Sociology*, vol. 31, no. 1, pp. 7–27.

Carvalho, M. J. (2003) *Entre as malhas do desvio* [*In the web of deviance*], Celta Editora, Oeiras.

Castel, R. (2003) *From Manual Workers to Wage Labourers: Transformation of the Social Question*, Transaction Publishers, New Brunswick.

Castro, J. (2009) 'Le tournant punitif. Y a-t-il des points de résistance? La réponse de l'expérience portugaise [*The punitive turn. Are there resistance points? The response of the Portuguese experience*]', *Déviance et Societé*, vol. 33, no. 3, pp. 295–313.

Cusson, M. (1974) *La resocialisation du jeune délinquant* [*The resocialization of young offenders*], Les Presses Universitaires de Montréal, Montréal.

DGRS (2008) *Difusão estatística 2007: volume 1* [Statistical information 2007: volume 1], Ministério da Justiça, Lisbon.

Feeley, M. M. & Simon, J. (1992) 'The new penology: notes on the emerging strategy of corrections and its implications', *Criminology*, vol. 30, no. 4, pp. 449–474.

Field, S. (2007) 'Practice cultures and the "new" youth justice in (England and) Wales', *British journal of criminology*, vol. 47, no. 2, pp. 311–330.

Fine, G. A. (1993) 'Ten lies of ethnography: moral dilemmas of field research', *Journal of Contemporary Ethnography*, vol. 22, no. 3, pp. 267–294.

Foucault, M. (1997) *Vigiar e punir* [*Discipline and punish: the birth of the prison*], Editora Vozes, Petrópolis.

Fox, K. J. (2005) 'Coercing change: how institutions induce correction in the culture of self-change', in *Ethnographies of Law and Social Control*, ed S. L. Burns, Elsevier, Amsterdam, pp. 105–119.

Francis, J., Kendrick, A. & Poso, T. (2007) 'On the margin? Residential child care in Scotland and Finland', *European Journal of Social Work*, vol. 10, no. 3, pp. 337–352.

Garland, D. (2001) *The Culture of Control*, Oxford University Press, Oxford.

Geertz, C. (1993) *The Interpretation of Cultures*, Fontana Press, London.

Goffman, E. (1971) *Asylums: Studies on the Social Situation of Mental Patients and Other Inmates*, Penguin Books, Middlesex.

Halsey, M. & Armitage, J. (2009) 'Incarcerating young people: the impact of custodial "care"', in *Youth Offending and Youth Justice*, eds M. Barry & F. McNeill, Jessica Kingsley Publishers, London, pp. 156–175.

Hammersley, M. & Atkinson, P. (1983) *Ethnography: Principles in Practice*, Tavistock Publications, London.

Henriksen, A., Degner, J. & Oscarsson, L. (2008) 'Youths in coercive residential care: attitudes towards key staff members' personal involvement, from a therapeutic alliance perspective', *European Journal of Social Work*, vol. 11, no. 2, pp. 145–159.

Houchins, D., Puckett-Patterson, D., Crosby, S., Shippen, M. E. & Jolivette, K. (2009) 'Barriers and facilitators to providing incarcerated youth with a quality education', *Preventing School Failure: Alternative Education for Children and Youth*, vol. 53, no. 3, pp. 159–166.

INE (2009) *50 anos de estatísticas da educação: volume 1* [*50 years of statistics in education: volume 1*], Gabinete de Estatística e Planeamento da Educação, Lisbon.

Jackson, S. (2010) 'Reconnecting care and education: from the Children Act 1989 to Care Matters', *Journal of Children's Services*, vol. 5, no. 3, pp. 48–61.

Kincheloe, J. L. & McLaren, P. L. (1998) 'Rethinking critical theory and qualitative research', in *The Landscape of Qualitative Research: Theories and Issues*, eds N. K. Denzin & Y. S. Lincoln, Sage, Thousand Oaks, CA, pp. 260–299.

Littlechild, B. (2008) 'Child protection social work: risks of fears and fears of risks – impossible tasks from impossible goals? *Social Policy and Administration*, vol. 42, no. 6, pp. 662–675.

Littlechild, B. (2009) 'Restorative justice, mediation and relational conflict resolution in work with young people in residential care', *Practice: Social Work in Action*, vol. 21, no. 4, pp. 229–240.

Lorenz, W. (2005) 'Social work and a new social order – challenging neo-liberalism's erosion of solidarity', *Social Work and Society*, vol. 3, no. 1, pp. 93–101.

Martin, P. Y. & Jackson, S. (2002) 'Educational success for children in public care: advice from a group of high achievers', *Child and Family Social Work*, vol. 7, no. 2, pp. 121–130.

Mathur, S. R. & Schoenfeld, N. (2010) 'Effective instructional practices in juvenile justice facilities: the need for effective instruction', *Behavioral Disorders*, vol. 36, no. 1, pp. 20–27.

Meeuwisse, A., & Swärd, H. (2007) 'Cross-national comparisons of social work: a question of initial assumptions and levels of analysis', *European Journal of Social Work*, vol. 10, no. 4, pp. 481–496.

Muncie, J. (2006) 'Governing young people: coherence and contradiction in contemporary youth justice', *Critical Social Policy*, vol. 26, no. 4, pp. 770–793.

Muncie, J. & Goldson, B. (2006) 'States of transition: convergence and diversity in international youth Justice', in *Comparative Youth Justice: Critical Issues*, eds J. Muncie & B. Goldson, Sage, London, pp. 196–218.

Muncie, J. & Hughes, G. (2004) 'Modes of youth governance: political rationalities, criminalization and resistance', in *Youth Justice: Critical Readings*, eds J. Muncie, G. Hughes & E. McLaughlin, Sage, London, pp. 1–18.

Neves, T. (2008) *Entre educativo e penitenciário* [*Between educational and penitentiary*], Afrontamento, Porto

Polsky, N. (1971) *Hustlers, Beats and Others*, Penguin Books, Harmondsworth.

Raine, J. W. & Willson, M. J. (1996) 'Managerialism and beyond: the case of criminal justice', *International Journal of Public Sector Management*, vol. 9, no. 4, pp. 20–33.

Rogowski, S. (2010) 'Young offending: towards a radical/critical social policy', *Journal of Youth Studies*, vol. 13, no. 2, pp. 197–211.

Santos, B. S. (1999) *Pela mão de Alice: o social e o político na pós-modernidade* [*Guided by Alice: the social and the political in post-modernity*], Afrontamento, Porto.

Singh, G. & Cowden, S. (2009) 'The social worker as intellectual', *European Journal of Social Work*, vol. 12, no. 4, pp. 479–493.

Stein, M. & Dixon, J. (2006) 'Young people leaving care in Scotland', *European Journal of Social Work*, vol. 9, no. 4, pp. 407–423.

Vacca, J. (2008) 'Crime can be prevented if schools teach juvenile offenders to read', *Children and Youth Services Review*, vol. 30, no. 9, pp. 1055–1062.

Van Maanen, J. (1988) *Tales of the Field: On Writing Ethnography*, University of Chicago Press, Chicago.

Wacquant, L. (2000) *As prisões da miséria* [*Prisons of poverty*], Celta Editora, Oeiras.

Wacquant, L. (2001) 'The penalisation of poverty and the rise of neo-liberalism', *European Journal on Criminal Policy and Research*, vol. 9, pp. 401–412.

Willis, P. & Trondman, M. (2000) 'Manifesto for ethnography', *Ethnography*, vol. 1, no. 1, pp. 5–16.

Action competence—a new trial aimed at social innovation in residential homes?

Handlekompetence—et nyt forsøg med sigte på social innovation i døgninstitutioner?

Niels Rosendal Jensen

This article reflects upon a project on Action Competence in Pedagogical Practice (ACP). The project developed and tested an intervention strategy in residential homes aimed at enhancing socially endangered children's life opportunities through learning and social inclusion. The ACP intervention was built upon a principle of 'soft' evidence-based practice and upon the premise that innovation based on research-generated knowledge and success with implementation strategies presupposed a linkage between professionals and researchers. The study of 200 children and young people in six residential homes was further based on an experimental design, prompting the participating institutions to change parts of their practice. Those changes were understood as social innovation which was at a later stage tested by the practitioners who worked with evidence-based knowledge about (1) socially endangered children (2) international research findings on intervention effects and (3) legislation plus a focus on three important factors: school, friendship and home. The article presents the intervention-model and its phases, its theoretical base and considers the methodological question, the barriers and eventually points to some interesting findings.

Artiklen reflekterer bl.a. teoretisk over HPA-projektet. Dette projekt udviklede og afprøvede en interventionsstrategi i døgninstitutioner med det mål at udvikle socialt udsatte børns livschancer gennem læring og social inklusion. HPA-interventionen byggede på et princip om 'blød' evidensbaseret praksis og tillige på den forudsætning, at innovation baseret på forskningsbaseret viden og succes med hensyn til implementeringsstrategier forudsatte en forbindelse mellem professionelle praktikere og forskere. Studiet af 200 børn og unge i 6 døgninstitutioner byggede endvidere på et eksperimentelt design, som søgte at fremme de deltagende institutioners muligheder for at ændre dele af deres praksisser. Ændringerne blev tolket som social innovation, der senere afprøvedes af de professionelle, som arbejdede ud fra evidensbaseret viden om (1) socialt udsatte børn, (2) internationale forskningsresultater om effekten af interventioner og (3) lovgivning plus fokus på 3 vigtige faktorer (skole, venskab og hjemlighed). Artiklen præsenterer interventionsmodellen og dens faser, dens teoretiske grundlag og inddrager det metodologiske spørgsmål, barriererne og peger afslutningsvist på nogle interessante fund.

Introduction

The article draws on a research project designed to investigate the implementation of a new approach to action competence development related to endangered children and youngsters. It focuses on the critical issue of how to transfer new knowledge from university to profession. Then, the theoretical framework upon which this study was anchored and the research methodology employed in this study are presented, while crucial questions of the research employed for this study are discussed. It further examines the issue of 'program intervention' and tries to reconstruct possible constraints. The article concludes with a short analysis of the findings from the study.

Socially Endangered Children—Theoretical End Empirical Background

The Action Competence in Pedagogical Practice (ACP) project takes its point of departure from theories of social heritage. We know that negative social heritage is linked both to socio-economic inequality *and* to problems of marginalisation and the difficulties that socially endangered children are exposed to. These two kinds of negative social heritage sometimes reinforce each other. It is difficult to break a marginalisation process once it has been set in motion—it is reproduced generation after generation, partly because of inadequate social networks and personal resources and competencies. Such processes are usually described as 'vicious circles'. Negative social heritage is defined as the situation whereby children from socially endangered families 'inherit', so to speak, the poorer chances in life connected with socially endangered or impoverished family conditions in an economic, cultural and social sense.

Research into social inequality, carried out by the 'grand old man' of Danish sociology of education (Hansen, 1982, 1995, 2003), shows that despite general economic prosperity, altered social conditions, greater social mobility but also increased social efforts towards better welfare for everyone in Denmark (Jørgensen et al., 1993; Jørgensen, 2002), it has not been possible to 'break the curve'; on the contrary, inequality seems to persist or in some forms, almost to have increased (cf. Petersen, 2008, 2009). In other words, it has not been possible to stop the negative social heritage defined here by the fact that the consequences of growing up under socially endangered conditions are transferred from generation to generation in the form of poorer economic, cultural and social chances in life. Research also shows that so-called 'pattern breakers', that is, people who do well against all odds, are characterised by upward social mobility and good cognitive and intellectual abilities. They are also characterised by doing well in and enjoying school and have supportive social resources behind them in the family, institutions and school.

Much research on social heritage primarily points to individual factors (divorce, long-term unemployment, etc.). But we searched for a structural perspective as well.

Therefore, the theoretical basis of the research project was inspired by Bourdieu's theory that social inequality evolves from the reproduction of power relationships and differences in the possibilities for social classes in positioning themselves (attaining a position) in society (Bourdieu, 1977, 1984, 1986; Bourdieu & Passeron, 1977). Such differences are connected with inequalities in human capital—that is, in addition to economic capital, also cultural capital, e.g. education, lifestyle and taste, and social capital, that is, networks, which give access to social resources and other people who can be drawn on for support in one's private life and work life. The three forms of capital are usually linked together in the concept of symbolic capital (Bourdieu, 1986; Jensen et al., 2005; Jensen, 2007). With reference to Bernstein's theories of the symbolic codes (Bernstein, 1973a, 1973b, 1977, 1990), it must additionally be assumed that institutions, schools and education risk contributing to the maintenance or even reinforcement of social inequality by a pedagogy often built upon the codes of the middle class. In other words, the forms of capital and competencies that are recognised in institutions and schools fit the values and beliefs of the middle class.

Children with different social and cultural backgrounds may, therefore, experience difficulties in interpreting these codes—they may not be familiar with them or they may be unable to use cultural tools (e.g. language), in such a way that their competencies are recognised.

Socially endangered groups may not be recognised for their competencies, but are instead assessed as 'incompetent', and the criteria used in the assessment are 'middle-class codes'. Moreover, growing up in a postmodern society characterised by rapid change, globalisation and new demands and challenges to the individual's competencies risk intensifying the problem of social inequality (Beck, 1992). Some social theorists claim that the new times give individuals new chances to create a new self, free of previous generations' restrictions (Giddens, 1990, 1991), while others

(Beck, 1992) claim on the contrary that a postmodern society implies new risks and that inequality is increased.

The project defines thus socially endangered children as children who are at risk or who are at risk of becoming excluded in institutions, schools and the educational system and later in society in general as a consequence of growing up under poor social conditions characterised by poverty, parental unemployment and lack of education, social insecurity and/or difficult divorces (Jensen, 2007). Such background conditions are evidenced to have a major impact on children's life opportunities by affecting their intellectual, linguistic and social competences. At the same time, those children are being marginalised and socially excluded in various societal arenas and institutions. As the theory of Bourdieu suggests, we may assume that belonging to one of society's less privileged or even underprivileged strata is passed on from generation to generation (Bourdieu, 1986), as it seems that social inequality is reproduced. Educational research and register-based generation studies show that despite great societal changes, globalisation and so-called new possibilities for all (Giddens, 1990, 1991), the hypothesis of reproduction still seems to be robust.On the basis of a Bourdieu-approach to the phenomena of social inequality outlined here, we lean towards the last-mentioned assumption that inequality is embedded in current social conditions and risks being augmented through increased polarisation between so-called 'competent' and 'incompetent' individuals. Consequently, these theoretical aspects of marginalisation in a world based on globalisation and new risks should inform our thinking about goals and methods in childhood and youth intervention strategies in the future.

It is not a 'piece of cake' to develop ways out for young people. Therefore, we planned to implement an intervention strategy based on the perspective of action competence. This statement is in no way breaking news, but to develop new practices demands a certain social innovation (cf. Nygren, 2004). Our thinking combined the approach of Bourdieu with that of competence development of children as well as professionals.

Methodology, Aims and Constraints

As already mentioned, we sought an intervention strategy, built upon the premise that innovation based on research-generated knowledge and success with implementation strategies presupposed the existence of a linkage between professionals and researchers and implications of learning and knowing processes for the professionals' work with innovation. This is the point where we find a *first serious problem or challenge*. The classical Welfare State is substituted by a mixtum compositum of welfare and competitive state (Hirsch, 1995; Jossop, 2002; Pedersen, 2011), which does not mean that the Welfare State and its universalistic principles are outdated. However, the competitive state does not aim towards equality or equal treatment. For example, it differentiates between those in work and those not. The first are worthy receivers of benefits, and the latter not. The ideal citizen today is seen as a person committed to work. The public servant has to consider how many public resources should be used to make persons fit for work.

First, parents are guided to help their children in school, aiming at providing their child with the competencies demanded in the labour market, that is, preparation for work. Second, transitions in work, aimed at helping people already having a job to shift from one workplace to another or from work to maternity leave or to further education. As a third example, resignation or retirement from work—the unemployed, the patient and the client are distributed by an officer in charge according to capacity for work or will to work. The willing ones are allocated to unemployment benefits and activation, whilst those not fit for work are placed in 'passive support'. The fourth example relates to out-of-work-positions—a situation defined by the fact that you are not part of the labour market.

What is the point? It is to emphasise the new conditions of being a young person in Denmark. Furthermore, the idea is to call attention to basic changes: 'efficiency' is substituted for professional judgement, meaning that the employee has to show consideration for the total situation of the institution or the budget of the municipality. The outcome is 'tailor-made solutions', an individual solution for each person weighing pros and cons: how many working hours am I capable of using in this case? How many resources should be used to urge this person to find a job? How do my considerations fit in with the budget of my institutions? Within the framework of a 'fluid organisation' this becomes even more difficult.

The second challenge is, having reflected upon the differences between research and theoretical work on the one hand and the practical work of social pedagogues on the other hand, that it struck me that we had to 'reconcile' two different cycles. The first could be labelled 'direct action', primarily related to the users, secondarily related to colleagues and their system of action and tertiarily related to other functional parts of systems (school, family background, etc.). The developmental dynamic takes place in a continuum of tensions between 'lifelong leaning' and 'the learning organisation'. This produces a cycle of locally situated action competence (Giddens, 1984; Nygren, 2004), which constitutes the transformation of knowledge in two main forms: development of competences and performance. To learn from experiences is to perform while observing and interpreting your own as well as your colleagues' contributions. Learning from experiences is thereby conditioned as a non-linear process due to the fact that goals, persons, fields, institutions, situations, plans and actors' feelings of control are all parts of social pedagogical practice. In addition, such processes are embedded in societal and cultural conditions, legislation, regulations and so on.

The second cycle derives from science. Scientific knowledge on social pedagogy has a marginal position in relation to the complexity of everyday work in institutions. This does not imply that such knowledge is superfluous. This reflection led me to present two working hypotheses: (1) Formation of professional action competence is a social process and thus dependent on the formation of a professional culture. An indicator of successful professionalisation must be observed as a professional habitus

(Bourdieu). (2) The difference between the system or cycle of science and that of practice shows that universities and universities of applied science cannot transfer professional action competence, but only communicate knowledge. However, education can provide students with tools for analysing, evaluating and reflecting practice. This further means that science and practice cooperate in a distinct way. Science commutes between basic research and action research, whilst practice commutes between routine and innovation. Practice needs action research when approximating innovation, e.g. an unsolved problem in daily practice. But while there is life there is hope—the reconciliation could be found in local developmental innovation supported by scientific knowledge (Jensen, 2008).

On the basis of these insights which became more obvious at the end of the project—the intervention drew upon the idea of the qualitative experiment inspired by Kleining (1986). He suggests six methods of intervention: separation/segmentation, combination, reduction, intensification, substitution and transformation. By offering these methods a broad range of experimental actions were presented. Let me use the relationship to school as an example. Social pedagogues were asked to intensify their relationship with the teachers at the local school in order to support or scaffold their 'inmates' in a better way than usual. This intervention meant that they had to develop cooperation on such issues as the children's homework and their own participation in evening meetings with other parents and so on. They also had to transform their view on schoolteachers, among other things 'bury the hatchet' between the two professions. Furthermore, some of the residential homes used the intensified cooperation to open the eyes and minds of all children by meeting in class and explaining what a modern residential home is. In addition, they opened their own doors at events like birthday celebrations to show that this was not a prison. Thereby they succeeded in supporting friendships between their own children and the home-based children in the class.

The qualitative experiment is like a never-ending story, you can intervene on many levels and in many fields and particularly support the competent, professional initiative at the local institution by handing over the idea of continuous experimenting (= social innovation). Hence, qualitative experiments will look like loose ends or to be more exact open a plethora of local options (bottom-up) within a common platform (top-down). We did not expect those loose ends to be tied up. On the contrary researchers and practitioners were supposed to meet in interplay to find the unity of diversity.

The project ran through five phases:

- *Phase 1.* Identification and clarification of existing knowledge about the target group, based on previous research, social and educational political documents and on the participating institutions' strategies for developing and improving pedagogical work in relation to socially endangered children; The Qualification material (October 2005 to September 2006).

- *Phase 2.* Development of an intervention strategy, based on a qualification package. This phase consisted of three elements: (1) process descriptions, (2) tools based on input and knowledge and (3) implementation strategy. Input was gathered from background papers from research groups, theoretical implementations and ideas about organisation development—in an action competence perspective. Planning and specification of the collaboration between researchers, centres for higher education and consultants and specialists from the municipalities (April 2006 to September 2006).
- *Phase 3.* Strategic selection of the residential homes. Six institutions were selected as intervention institutions and a board of practical experts in the field as a reference group. In total this comprises approximately 100–200 children, 7–18 years of age (May 2006 to August 2006).
- *Phase 4.* Implementation of the intervention. Observations in the selected residential homes (starting September 2006 to May 2008)—and later revised due to temporary displacement.
- *Phase 5.* Effect-analyses. First baseline assessments. A database was established and the first competence assessments were conducted in the institutions, making the first comparisons between intervention institutions possible. Along with continuous observations and qualitative interviews in the institutions, midway and final assessments were conducted. Furthermore, data about pedagogical processes were collected (September 2006 to May 2009).

As to the time frame, the baseline assessments on children's competences were carried out in September 2006; the second assessment was made in May 2007 and the third took place in May 2008 around the time of finishing the intervention. We were trying to get permission to follow a single institution even further and also to continue an intervention more intensively after May 2008 but this proved impossible due to organisational changes.

In the year 2004, about 8000 children and youngsters were placed in residential institutions (traditional residential homes and more family-like homes, but not foster care). Foster care is a dominant form of placement, but our interest focused on public and private residential homes, representing about 30% (2500) of children and young persons aged between 7 and 14 years who were placed outside their own home (Danmarks Statistik, 2004).

The six residential homes selected were characterised by:

- Having a stable staff of educated pedagogues—unlike many residential homes which have a majority of unskilled employees.
- Having a 'youth milieu', meaning that the number of youngsters accommodated in each setting should be more than 10.
- Including treatment only for youngsters with problems of social interaction [excluding institutions marked by other reasons for placing young people in care (e.g. a medical diagnosis)]

- Institutions situated in the Copenhagen and Aarhus area.
- Institutions characterised as exemplifying 'good practice' by a board of out-standing leaders within the field.
- Institutions that wanted to participate voluntarily.

Although these criteria seem easily achievable it turned out to be much more difficult than expected to find homes that met our requirements. The whole field is 'overcrowded' by projects, meaning that the density of ongoing projects (ordered by the municipality or region, decided voluntarily or seen as a way to get more resources, etc.) is heavy. One of the institutions felt it was 'chosen' and had its own agenda, aiming at showing that social pedagogy works and good results are achieved. Many negotiations had to be carried out before the final selection of participating institutions. When institutions feel crowded by a large number of ongoing projects they have to fit our project into the existing ones. This is *the third serious problem*. It meant picking up what fitted in and dropping parts of our project that did not. The implementation was constrained by such unavoidable deviations from the original project plan.

The aims were to enhance new perspectives on school, friendship and home. The institutions were supposed to work with 'the whole package', but were free to choose their own point of departure, based on the analysis of the gap between what professionals thought they did, and what children and youngsters thought. Those foci were based on state-of-the-art Danish, Nordic and some international research (Nielsen, 2006). The 'blind spots' in Danish residential homes proved to be a lack of systematic support for children at school, too little attention to establishing friendships and networks outside the home (e.g. sports clubs, hobbies and other organisations for children of the same age) and recognising the importance of the residential home as the children and youngsters' other home.

This brings us to *the fourth problem or challenge*. Pedagogues are characterised by a conviction of indispensability. They are convinced of being the most important persons in a given child's or youngster's life. They act as substitutes to parents. Parents have done so and so wrong, now it is time to say good bye and take responsibility for the children. This attitude is basically false, and when testing it against empirical data, it becomes obvious that children and youngsters are much more dependent on their biological parents and their peers than on the adult pedagogues. A certain pecking order emerges among children and youngsters which the staff are not able to control. The old proverb hits it on the nail: 'when the cat's away, the mice will play'. During the day time adults try to control and regulate social attitudes and patterns. But at late evenings or over the weekend children and youngsters are competing to get a better position in their own hierarchy. Research shows the importance of physical strength or impudence towards the staff as criteria for inclusion in the group of peers. Peer relationships seem to lead to a 'danger of infection', meaning that children and young persons placed outside their home easily get into bad company. They are in many ways excluded and often challenge the rules;

they are forced to find friends among the other 'inmates', and the bad boys and girls are usually the dominant ones (Egelund *et al.*, 2010).

To sum up: the general changes of institutions, the existence of two cycles, the troubles of overcrowded institutions and the overestimation of pedagogical influence on the children and youngsters had to be taken into account to prevent future problems in the implementation of the project.

Intervention Studies

International research seems to indicate that positive results in relation to socially endangered children and youngsters can be achieved by early intervention. Such interventions are characterised by a goal-oriented effort towards stimulating at-risk children's cognitive abilities, well-being and health in a broad sense. However, these studies do not shed light on the cultural and social aspects of visible and invisible processes of exclusion in the educational environment that influence the intended outcomes of initiatives and interventions.

It is, moreover, evident that research is characterised by great variations in definitions of socially endangered children. The target groups are often 'taken-for-granted', even though we know they cover many different sub-groups of children or youngsters at risk, for example, children from vulnerable families, or living in poverty, or whose parents lack education and cultural and social competences. In terms of interventions, we are able to identify a progression from early American Randomized Controlled Trial (RCT) studies whose designs were constructed as very strict experimental interventions and assessments aimed at measuring effects on children's cognitive skills, development and behaviour (Jespersen, 2006; Jensen, 2007) towards new longitudinal studies which examine effects of different kinds of state care (Langager, 2006; Nielsen, 2006).

In research, two paradigms have been identified up to now: (1) a compensation strategy (or so-called 'blaming the victim' strategy)—socially endangered children 'lack' something which they need to be compensated for and (2) an innovation strategy aiming at promoting socially endangered children's life opportunities through education, competence development and social inclusion.

The Intervention Programme

The purpose of the intervention and effect study presented here is two-sided: on the one hand, it aims at developing and testing an intervention strategy which originates in the innovation paradigm, and on the other hand it aims at examining the effects. The question is 'what are the effects of an intervention aimed at social innovation in relation to socially endangered children's competence development and what factors promote/restrict effects?'

The intervention strategy was developed and inspired by research into implementation and working life. This was translated into the ACP vision of making 'bottom-up' and 'top-down' perspectives meet. Obviously many conflicts of interests, poor local conditions or traditions, ideologies and so on did in fact oppose a successful intervention. We intended to examine the latter field, which in terms of research is not much explored, by using knowledge about the status of the institutions concerning various factors which are assumed to be of importance in working innovatively (organisation, level of education of staff, working conditions, etc.). The intervention showed that for professionals, the most important single factor seemed to be 'control over own working situation'.

The intervention was based upon a principle of 'soft' evidence-based practice—that is, innovation based on knowledge from selected research. The ACP-project's approach to evidence-based practice is embedded in theories of science, which assume that practice will change if a user perspective, that is, involvement of participants and ownership, becomes central (Sommerfeld, 2005). Furthermore, implementation research (Winter & Nielsen, 2008), theories on culture from a communication perspective and innovation research in working life (e.g. Høyrup & Elkjaer, 2006) have documented that a plethora of other circumstances related to the processes of learning and knowing in work organisations can either restrict or promote an innovation and influence its effectiveness.

The strategy was based on material developed by the researchers—a so-called qualification package—that presented evidence-based knowledge about (1) socially endangered children, background variables, the concept of action competence, (2) effects of intervention based on international research and contra-indicative effects in relation to exclusion and (3) legislation in the field (educational learning plans and action plans in residential institutions). The evidence-based knowledge from these three areas was merged with a fourth field of knowledge, practitioners' knowledge, consisting partly of explicit and implicit experiences from practice, partly of theoretical knowledge and common knowledge in the institution. These elements interacted with evidence-based 'external' knowledge in selected strategic fields (Schön, 1983). The exchange of these different fields of knowledge was communicated through written material (an ACP 'portfolio'), through analyses of the gap between pedagogues' experiences of their own competences and children's competences ('GAP-profiles') and through local support and the facilitation of processes via consultants and courses, arranged and prepared by researchers. The implementation of knowledge converted into a new practice furthermore demands a connection between user and research perspectives. Our intervention intended to build upon and try to capture knowledge needs of the professionals, and their need for attaining ownership of their own developmental processes and interests.

The intervention consisted of a 'qualification package' addressed to the professionals, described and defined in advance, which comprises three elements: (1) a qualification folder—material built on evidence-based knowledge; (2) a competence development process—built on pedagogues' identification of their own competences and their qualifications for approaching the work in new ways and implementation processes; (3) specification of working with the ACP package and focus on local development models which had been adapted to local conditions and backgrounds:

- *The qualification folder—knowledge as a basis for action and change.* The qualification folder contained three fields of knowledge that were to be brought into interaction with a fourth, practical knowledge. The fields of knowledge selected are all based on research results on the action competence perspective (the individual field of knowledge), exclusion processes (the institutional field of knowledge) and the legal basis (the political field of knowledge). Pedagogues' knowledge and experience (the practical field of knowledge) is the fourth field, and the whole idea behind the intervention was that the fourth field of knowledge was brought into interaction with the three other fields of knowledge.

- *Competence development and professionals' learning processes start with gap analyses.* The gap between what pedagogues believed they supported and what real competences children and youngsters demonstrated was identified using statistical analyses, and a local profile of the gap in a whole institution was delivered to the institutions. On the basis of this identification, the institution described and set its own new goals for working with the children. The new goals had partly to answer the results of the gap, and partly the knowledge generated from the study part of the folder. This gap was analysed once in the process—the institutions then began to set their own goals on the common basis presented in the whole intervention package.

- *Implementation processes.* The management and organisation was planned in cooperation with the research group and consultants and was carried out throughout the entire intervention period (2006—May 2008). The implementation strategy started with (1) introductory days for everyone involved, (2) a two-day course for consultants and (3) a course for heads of institutions. The study part of the folder was begun right before the introductory days, not run by us, but by the heads of the institutions themselves, with the support of consultants. How the implementation strategy was planned and carried out was decided in the institutions and the implementation process ran over a period of a year and a half.

Throughout the whole intervention (2006–2008), institutions and municipalities were given the opportunity to invite researchers and consultants to help them initiate and support the process depending on what needs they might gradually experience and to discuss the contents of the qualification material, the 'portfolio' and the GAP-analyses, translated into their actual practice. Furthermore, the researchers held regular network meetings with the coordinating groups, which consisted of consultants from centres for further education and practitioners, aiming at discussing the course of the processes and possible changes or difficulties that they faced on their way. The practitioners were also invited to join 'café evenings' where researchers gave lectures on selected topics such as socially endangered children, learning, curriculum, inclusion and exclusion, innovation and so on, aiming at establishing a connection between research and practice.

Instead of being controlled solely by methods, the intervention is both governed by theory and goals and is targeted at a joint overall aim: pedagogues have to develop their practice through their own competence analysis and practice analysis. The disadvantage of working on the basis of an open innovation design is that the assessment of effect has to take into account that the method is carried out locally and, therefore, includes variations of the ACP vision. Overcoming this dilemma is not an easy task, but by drawing on and using data—in addition to the effect assessment—on the local processes, that is, institutional conditions, educational processes and the pedagogues' competence development and their descriptions of knowledge and learning processes, much of that problem came 'under control'.

Social Innovation

Innovation is not identical to intervention, the main difference being that innovation covers the whole process from a new idea to a realised product or procedure (Swedberg, 2009). Basically, innovation is related to change and the emergence of something new. Social innovation is manifested in the professionals' work with the programme's goal-based and theory-based perspectives aiming at a concrete product/ effect, namely socially endangered children's competence development through learning and social inclusion.

The project's overall value foundation is a so-called 'involvement of the agent perspective', that is, that the intervention process focused on (1) involving the agents' ownership and possibilities of entering a dialogue about their assignment, (2) ensuring that the agents think the project makes sense, that is, that it matches their needs for new methods, their previous experiences and need for developing their own practices and (3) ensuring that it will be possible to attain a common language and time to translate new knowledge into practice. A focus on reflective action and cooperation between the participating agents, that is, between researchers, consultants and practitioners, was considered crucial while the ACP-programme was being created (see e.g. Gould & Baldwin, 2004; Boud *et al.*, 2006; Fook & Gardner, 2007).

We initiated and analysed the possibilities of a social innovation from three perspectives.

A 'Communication and Culture' Theoretical Perspective

The local culture of an institution reflects itself in specific communication practices, and such practices control and regulate the use or non-use of knowledge among staff members. To paraphrase Bourdieu, a doxa is established due to professional education and institutional culture which implies a certain kind of reserve concerning new knowledge.

A System Theoretical Perspective

The challenge was not only comprised of conflicts of interest, therefore, but also it became necessary to supplement the above perspective with systems theory, according to which the various agents participating in the project perceive of the project and their roles differently, depending on their job function and the kind of communication culture they are a part of.

An Implementation and Network Theoretical Perspective

The relation between the various actors and the interplay between them would be of great importance to the exchanges taking place and to the entire implementation process. New possibilities were within range—however, the agents also met new demands. Consequently, we listened to all agent groups to examine what new tools they thought had become available to them and the problems they encountered.

We observed a successful innovation to be built upon:

- an innovative culture emphasising the professionals' knowledge, competences and implementation strategies;
- a working and learning environment that stresses dialogue, reflection and creativity;
- ownership and systematic testing of ideas in a joint renewal of practice.

Effects of ACP Intervention—Methods and Materials

The ACP-project (at least the part on residential homes) looked for new ways in experimentally designed intervention and effect studies, thus looking for a combination of a stringent evidence concept, where the method was tested and effects were established, and an open principle in order to attain knowledge about the contextualisation of the effects. The interventions were thoroughly described and based on the assumption that local innovation produced the best effect. The design itself made it possible to examine differences in the way in which the ACP intervention was carried out in practice.

The study of the six selected institutions examined how socially endangered children's social and learning competences were influenced by the goal-oriented ACP intervention, which aims at (1) enhancing children's competences, (2) identifying and preventing potential exclusion processes (within the residential home as well as in the local environment). The children's social background was identified through visits made by the administrations of the residential homes.

Effects were measured 'in relation to' children's learning and competence development, which we found to be indicative of a functioning intervention aimed at children's learning and social development (the individual level), not measured 'on' children's development, since the aim of this part of the project was to get a clearer understanding of how pedagogues were developing competencies. This meant that the three focal points below had to do with changed or new actions on the part of the social pedagogues:

- *How are the institutions supporting children's learning possibilities/school* (competence development). Pedagogues were asked to be particularly aware that children in residential homes are usually met with reservation by schoolteachers in the outside environment. The project emphasised that pedagogues should take responsibility for assisting children in doing their homework and so on.
- *How institutions are supporting children's socio-emotional competence/friendship*—this was organised in terms of friendship or networking, e.g. by emphasising the development of social adjustment, social skills, identity, ability to take control, identity development and self-esteem and social understanding/readiness. The intention was that pedagogues should address this question very seriously, since research showed that children who had been 'put away' in residential homes were on average found to be unable to build stable and lasting contacts, meaning that they eventually became isolated.
- *How institutions enable children to feel that the residential setting is their home*—recent research in Denmark pointed to the importance of getting children in residential homes to 'feel at home'; therefore, we asked what the institutions were doing to make being 'out-of-home' as similar as possible to 'being-at-home'.

The assessment of innovation processes (institutional level) was based upon descriptions of institutions which were carried out in 2006–2007—as a kind of baseline assessment or starting point. Subsequently, we used the conditions for innovation in the analysis model and follow-up intensive data collections were planned in selected institutions—selected in the sense that the institutions could decide which spokespeople (leaders and social pedagogues) should participate in a broad qualitative interview.

Both pedagogues and parents acted as informants about the children's competencies. The outcomes were controlled in relation to background variables, including socio-economic conditions, cultural/educational conditions, relation/linking to the labour market, risk events in the family, and family and social events, such as divorce or death. The results were controlled further in relation to conditions that might hamper intervention, mechanisms in the institutions related to structural conditions, pedagogic conditions, readiness to engage in development/innovation and implementation strategies, but also mechanisms related to the external framework, municipal conditions, events, reorganisations, mergers and other development trends as well as other factors stemming from a postmodern world characterised by turbulence, complexity and rapid change. The municipalities' other strategies, continuing/further education and the educational level of pre-school teachers, innovation strategies and so on were parts of the assessment.

A New Design—Goals-Orientation

The ACP programme represented in principle a contribution to the development of new, mixed methods designs, from a method-oriented design to a goal- and theory-oriented design with a focus on staff-driven innovation. Uncontrollable aspects of the controlled design were, therefore, allowed and were used constructively, that is, they were used in the analysis aiming at identification of indicators of 'good practice'—seen in the perspective of innovation.

The methodological challenge consisted in collecting data which made it possible to identify 'good practice' in the innovation, that is, the data collection had to aim at effects at the level of pedagogues' competences as well as social innovation. The latter was examined by using descriptions of institutions as baseline and final assessments, focusing on factors which are assumed to support strategies, a working and learning environment that enhances dialogue, reflection, creativity and ownership and systematic testing of ideas in a joint renewal of practice. We attempted to solve this methodological problem by structuring the analysis around the above-mentioned three theoretical perspectives focusing on social innovation: implementation and network theory, system theory and theories on culture from a communication perspective.

Furthermore, it became relevant to 'fill out the gap' with theories of governance in order to understand the significance of participation and ownership, and eventually, the question of evidence was treated as a specific analytical perspective—also aiming at looking at possibilities and change potentials through a social innovation, like the one the ACP programme was initiating and testing.

Conclusion

The intervention succeeded in sharpening the focus on school, friendship and home. Interviews showed that pedagogues gave more attention to these three issues. The qualification folder was studied, discussed and related to own experiences. Collective reflection on efforts and outcomes became part of everyday practice, at least during the intervention. At least one of the six institutions focused intensively on school and found a valuable way of supporting children by hiring a part time schoolteacher (Jensen, 2009).

Of course, pedagogues do not swallow everything you tell them—research based or not. They have to digest the message comfortably, discuss it with colleagues and look for links between the qualification folder and their own experiences and show a general readiness to acquire new knowledge and new methods. This takes time, and in modern or fluid organisations the staff's time is also administrative time, meaning that study circles or study work in relation to the qualification folder became 'contested terrain'.

When the main substance of the whole idea is accepted, organising takes over. Evidence shows that one or two pedagogues had to be responsible for the implementation of the project, while leaders had to protect the implementation of the project from being overruled by many other and necessary activities. An unanticipated radical reform of municipality structure occurred in 2006/2007, changing organisational structures, tasks and target groups for more institutions.

Staff experienced those changes as a 'state of emergency' and felt everyday routines disappear. All six institutions met severe problems—notably high staff turnover, meaning that the project almost had to start over again. This harmed the continuity of the whole project, and earlier experiences did not get a foothold. This partly meant a constraint on accumulation of practical experiences over the 3 years. The project was to some extent pervasive, but never ubiquitous in the daily practice of the social pedagogues involved.

References

Beck, U. (1992) *Risk Society: Towards a New Modernity*, SAGE, London.

Bernstein, B. (1973a) *Class, Codes and Control*, Vol. 1, Routledge & Kegan Paul, London.

Bernstein, B. (1973b) *Class, Codes and Control*, Vol. 2, Routledge & Kegan Paul, London.

Bernstein, B. (1977) *Class, Codes and Control*, Vol. 3, Routledge & Kegan Paul, London.

Bernstein, B. (1990) *Class, Codes and Control, vol. 4: The Structuring of Pedagogic Discourse*, Routledge, London.

Boud, D., Cressey, P. & Docherty, P. (eds) (2006) *Productive Reflection at Work: Learning for Changing Organizations*, Routledge, London and New York.

Bourdieu, P. (1977) 'Cultural reproduction and social reproduction', in *Power and Ideology in Education*, eds J. Karabel & A. H. Halsey, Oxford University Press, New York, pp. 487–511.

Bourdieu, P. (1984 [1979]) *Distinction: A Social Critique of the Judgment of Taste*. Richard Nice (tr.), Harvard University Press, Cambridge, MA.

Bourdieu, P. (1986) 'The forms of capital', in *Handbook of Theory and Research for the Sociology of Education*, ed. J. G. Richardson, Greenwood Press, New York, pp. 241–258.

Bourdieu, P. & Passeron, J.-C. (1977 [1970]) *Reproduction in Education, Society and Culture*. Richard Nice (tr.), Sage Publications, London.

Danmarks Statistik. (2004) 'Children and young persons placed outside of own home by region, place of accomodation, age and sex', *Statistikbanken (BIS2)*, [online] Available at: www.statbank.dk

Egelund, T., Jakobsen, T. B., Hammen, I., Olsson, M. & A. Høst (2010) *Sammenbrud i anbringelser af børn og unge: Erfaringer, forklaringer og årsagerne bag* [*Breakdown in placements of children and young persons: experiences, explanations, and causes behind*], SFI, København.

Fook, J. & Gardner, F. (2007) *Practising Critical Reflection: A Resource Handbook*, Open University Press/McGraw-Hill Education, Maidenhead.

Giddens, A. (1984) *The Constitution of Society: Introduction if the Theory of Structuration*, Polity Press, Oxford.

Giddens, A. (1990) *The Consequences of Modernity*, Stanford University Press, Stanford, CA.

Giddens, A. (1991) *Modernity and Self-Identity: Self and Society in the Late Modern Age*, Polity, Oxford.

Gould, N. & Baldwin, M. (eds) (2004) *Social Work, Critical Reflection and the Learning Organization*, Ashgate, Aldershot.

Hansen, E. J. (1982) *Hvem bryder den sociale arv?* [*Who is breaking the social heritage?*]. Socialforskningsinstituttet, København. Publikation 112.

Hansen, E. J. (1995) *En generation blev voksen* [*A generation grew up*], Socialforskningsinstituttet, København. Rapport 95:8.

Hansen, E. J. (2003) *Uddannelsessystemerne i sociologisk perspektiv,*. Hans Reitzels Forlag, København.

Hirsch, J. (1995) *Wettbewerbsstaat: Staat, Demokratie ind Politik im globalen Kapitalismus*, Edition ID-Archiv, Amsterdam and Berlin.

Høyrup, S. & Elkjaer, B. (2006) 'Reflection: taking it beyond the individual', in *Productive Reflection at Work*, eds D. Boud, P. Cressey & P. Docherty, Routledge, London and New York.

Jensen, B. (2005) *Kan daginstitutioner gøre en forskel? En undersøgelse af daginstitutioner og social arv* [*Can day care institutions make a difference? An inquiry into day care institutions and social heritage*], Socialforskningsinstituttet, København.

Jensen, B. (2007) *Social arv, pædagogik og læring i daginstitutioner* [*Social heritage, pedagogy and learning in the day care institution*], Hans Reitzels Forlag, København.

Jensen, B., Jensen, N. R., & Andersen, T. V. (2005) *Kompetence- og metodeudvikling i daginstitutioner—Om implementering af "ny" viden i praksis* [*Development of competence and method in day care institutions: on implementation of "New" knowledge in practice*], Danmarks Pædagogiske, Universitetsforlag, København.

Jensen, N. R. (2008) 'Forskning og udvikling—det moderne "hvide snit" mellem disciplin og profession? [*Research and development—the modern "lobotomy" between discipline and profession*]' in *Tidsskrift for Socialpædagogik*, eds Jan Jaap Routhuizen & Ullrich Rudenko Zeitler, VIAUC, Aarhus, vol. 21, pp. 22–31.

Jensen, N. R. (2009) *Handlekompetence i socialpædagogisk arbejde på døgninstitutioner* [*Competence of action in social pedagogical work in residential homes*]. København, Available at: www.dpu.dk/hpa/publikationer.

Jespersen, C. (2006) 'Socialt udsatte børn i dagtilbud', *Socialforskningsinstituttet*, vol. 6, p. 21.

Jørgensen, P. S. (2002) 'Risikobørn i Danmark', *Tidsskriftet Social Kritik*, vol. 84, pp. 98–110.

Jørgensen, P. S. et al. (1993) 'Risikobørn, hvem er de, hvad gør vi? [Children at risk, who are they, what do we do?]', *Udarbejdet for det tværministerielle børneudvalg* [*Reported for the cross-ministerial commission on children*], The Ministry of Social Affairs, Copenhagen, December 1993.

Jossop, B. (2002) *The Future of the Capitalist State*, Polity Press, Cambridge.

Kleining, G. (1986) 'Das qualitative experiment', *Kölner Zeitschrift für Soziologie und Sozialpsychologie*, vol. 38, pp. 724–750.

Langager, S. (2006) *Socialpædagogisk arbejde på døgninstitutioner/opholdssteder med særligt henblik på at udvikle handlekompetence* [*Social pedagogical work in residential homes with particular reference to developing competence of action*], Danmarks Pædagogiske Universitets Forlagøbenhavn, København, Available at: www.dpu.dk/hpa/publikationer.

Nielsen, H. S. (2006) *Indsats og virkning på døgninstitutioner for børn og unge: et litteraturreview* [*Effort and effect in residential homes for children and young persons: a review of literature*], Danmarks Pædagogiske Universitets Forlag, København.

Nygren, P. (2004) *Handlingskompetanse: Om profesjonelle mennesker* [*Competence of action: about professional people*], Gyldendal Akademisk, Oslo.

Pedersen, O. K. (2011) *Konkurrencestaten* [*The competitive state*], Hans Reitzels Forlag, København.

Petersen, K. E. (2008) 'Working with socially endangered children in Danish Day-care institutions', *International Social Work & Society News Magazine*, Available at: www.socmag.net

Petersen, K. E. (2009) *Omsorg for socialt udsatte børn. En analyse af pædagogers kompetencer og pædagogiske arbejde med socialt udsatte børn i daginstitutioner*, Ph.D.-afhandling, Institut for Pædagogik, DPU, Aarhus.

Schön, D. (1983) *The Reflective Practitioner: How Professionals think in Action*, Temple, London.

Sommerfeld, P. (ed.) (2005) *Evidence-Based Social Work: Towards a New Professionalism*. Peter Lang, Bern, Berlin, Frankfurt am Main, New York, Oxford and Wien.

Swedberg, R. (2009) 'Schumpeter's full model of entrepreneurship: economic, non-economic and social entrepreneurship', in *An Introduction to Social Entrepreneurship: Voices, Preconditions, Contexts*, ed. R. Ziegler, Edward Elgar, Cheltenham and Northampton.

Winter, S. C. & Nielsen, V. L. (2008) *Implementering af politik* [*Implementation of politics*], Hans Reitzels Forlag, København.

The relevance and experience of education from the perspective of Croatian youth in-care

Iskustva i značaj obrazovanja iz perspektive mladih u javnoj skrbi u Hrvatskoj

Branka Sladović Franz & Vanja Branica

Education can contribute to the well-being of children and youth in out-of-home care by increasing resilience, acting as a secure base and enhancing life chances and pathways. This paper presents results of a qualitative study which aimed to examine the educational opportunities of youth in public care in Croatia from the user's perspective. A brief review of Croatian experience regarding in-care youth is presented and discussed. Six focus groups were conducted with 31 youth from children's homes and foster families. Participants perceive education as important for all children and youth because it can enable better life conditions and improve employment possibilities but they consider it to be even more important for in-care children due to their lack of a stable family base, financial insecurity and pressure to be independent. Educational experiences reveal different educational choices, circumstances that promote and those that impede education, as well as a differentiated approach to in-care children. The young people pointed to several factors that facilitate positive educational outcome: personal strengths and self-efficacy, financial support and a good relationship with professionals.

Obrazovanje može pridonijeti dobrobiti djece i mladih u javnoj skrbi povećavajući njihovu otpornost, njihove životne mogućnosti te djelujući kao sigurno mjesto. U ovom su radu prikazani rezultati istraživanja provedenog s ciljem upoznavanja obrazovnih mogućnosti mladih u javnoj skrbi u Hrvatskoj iz korisničke perspektive. Kratko je prikazan pregled hrvatskih iskustava u svezi mladih u javnoj skrbi. Provedeno je šest fokus grupa u kojoj je sudjelovala 31 mlada osoba smještena u institucionalni ili udomiteljski smještaj. Sudionici su percipirali obrazovanje ili jednako važnim za svu djecu i mlade jer osigurava bolje životne uvjete i poboljšava mogućnosti zaposlenja ili ga smatraju čak i važnijim za djecu u javnoj skrbi s obzirom da njima nedostaje stabilno obiteljsko utočište, financijska sigurnost te osjećaju pritisak da moraju biti samostalni. Edukacijska iskustva otkrivaju i da su donijeli različite obrazovne izbore, no i da su bili suočeni s okolnostima koje unaprjeduju ali i onima koje otežavaju njihovo obrazovanje kao i da su doživjeli različito ponašanje prema njima koji dolaze iz javne skrbi u odnosu na ostale vršnjake. Mladi su ukazali na nekoliko čimbenika koji promoviraju bolji obrazovni ishod: osobne snage i učinkovitost, financijska podrška i odnos sa stručnjacima.

Introduction

Child welfare in Croatia is grounded in legislation, which is in accordance with the United Nations Convention on the Rights of the Child and the principle of the child's best interest. The main shortcoming is the lack of early intervention and family support programmes in local communities, especially in rural areas (Ajduković, 2008). From the beginning of twentieth century two dominant types of out-of-home care developed: institutional and foster home placement. In the year 2010, children's homes in Croatia provided placement for 1017 children without adequate parental care and there were 2001 children living in 1216 foster families. Most of the children are of compulsory school age (Ministry of Health and Social Welfare Croatia, 2010). In recent years, there has been a slow process of deinstitutionalisation with more emphasis on fostering and downsizing of children's homes. There are also some small housing units where between three and five young people live together under the supervision of a care worker with the purpose of preparing them to leave the care system and live independently. This option is only available to older youth.

The most frequent reasons for out-of-home placement in Croatia are child abuse and neglect, disturbed family relations, abandonment and poverty (although the last is rarely the only reason) (Ajduković, 2004). This is in accordance with findings in other central and eastern European countries (Gudbrandsson, 2003). Longitudinal research on the psychosocial functioning of children in public care in Croatia (2000–2005) showed that children are entering public care when they are aged seven years on average, and typically stay in care for about four years (Ajduković & Sladović

Franz, 2005). The academic achievement of children in care was found to be generally low. However, an important finding was that their behavioural and emotional problems were significantly more related to their current situation and circumstances and the general level of experienced everyday stress rather than unfavourable life circumstances prior to placement (Ajduković & Sladović Franz, 2005). Significant sources of stress were problems in adjustment to school, poor school performance and perception of less social support (Sladović Franz, 2004). Results showed that fostered children adjusted better to school, and had better school attainment than children in residential care (Kregar Orešković & Rajhvajn, 2007).

Education in Croatia is still dominantly state organised and officially available to everyone with good grades. Elementary school lasts for eight years and is obligatory, while secondary school, not compulsory, is for three or four years depending on programmes. Higher education is in accordance with the Bologna process in terms of mobility and course credits transferable to other European countries. Public higher education is free for students, who achieve a certain standard, while those who are less successful may be supported by their families. Higher education is hard to access for children in public care due to earlier lower academic achievement and lack of financial and other kinds of support, which are only available for a few of the very best students. At the moment there are 15 of them financed by the Ministry of Health and Social Welfare and 61 more received scholarships from donor organisations in 2008–2010. Some measures aiming to improve conditions for in-care students have emerged lately: for example, youth can stay longer at independent units or can get placement at student dormitories. Some non-profit humanitarian agencies are providing scholarships, publishing brochures, organising donor events or advocating for funds through public media, websites and social networks.

Research in other European countries shows that the majority of children in care have a much reduced chance of progressing to higher education (Jackson & Cameron, 2012). In Sweden, Vinnerljung et al. (2005) found that children growing up in public care have a three times higher risk of entering adulthood with only basic education. There is no comparable quantitative research in Croatia but the situation appears to be similar. Many children are coming into public care with educational shortcomings which often represent the basis for numerous further causes of lower educational attainment, such as school exclusion, low expectations on the part of children themselves, their care workers and teachers, inadequate planning and support and lack of attention by social workers to educational needs (cf. Francis, 2000). The contention of the present paper is that, in Croatia low attainment and marginalisation of education have been a normal part of growing up in public care for far too long.

Whatever the reasons for academic difficulties, more importance should be given to ways to overcome them. Good academic achievement should be aimed for because it supports personal resilience and social inclusion and acts as an important protective factor (Jackson, 2007). As Gilligan has argued, school provides opportunities for creating positive relations with peers and teachers, helps to develop better self-esteem and can act as a complementary secure base (Gilligan, 1998 quoted by Dent & Cameron, 2003). In-care youth have a strong need for normalisation, to receive positive encouragement and to have a good relationship with a social worker, who should show genuine concern for their welfare, enhance their educational opportunities and must also serve as a liaison to out-of-care future life (Martin & Jackson, 2002). In Croatia, as in other countries (Dent & Cameron, 2003, Jackson, 2007), it seems that social work practice in general is focused on child and home issues and that there is a lack of concern for children's perspectives and interdisciplinary cooperation in securing children's rights and well-being.

Education has a significant role for all children and is always stressed as a very important factor by the adults. It has been pointed out as one of the priorities in numerous documents and social welfare development strategies as a way to overcome social exclusion of vulnerable groups, particularly children in public care—see for example, the Croatian national activity plan for children's rights and interests 2006–2012 (Ministry of Family, Veteran's Affairs and Intergenerational Solidarity, 2006). However, it seems that not enough research work has been conducted to find out how children and youth in the public care perceive education and whether education is really important to them. What are their motives for trying to do well at school and to have higher aspirations and ambitions? Research in other countries has shown that young people's personal motivation and attitudes are a crucial element in raising educational achievement (Korintus et al., 2010). It is therefore, our goal in this paper to explore the young people's own perception of the role, possibilities and relevance of education in their lives, to find out how they describe their educational experiences and what they think promotes a positive educational outcome, so that discussion and actions within the social work profession can move in a direction that supports resilience instead of reinforcing disadvantage and unequal opportunities.

Procedure and Sample

In-care youth can be seen as 'experts by experience'; they have the potential to give professionals an insight into educational possibilities from the user's perspective, which should be used for discussion and development of practice. In order to get an in-depth understanding of the perspective of youth in care on education, we have chosen the qualitative method as a way to obtain subjective viewpoints of participants and gain new information (Flick et al., 2004). This is a new approach to research on the issue in Croatia and the first attempt to look at the current situation from the viewpoint of those most closely concerned.

The study is based on focus groups, because we hoped to gain insight into commonalities and differences in viewpoints of youth and also to hear their experience and attitudes. The research participants consisted of 31 youths living in public care, 17 girls and 14 boys. The majority of youths (21/31), were aged 17 and 18 years old, mostly attending vocational secondary school, training for occupations such as cosmetics, plumbing, etc. (14). Only four attended grammar (academic secondary) school; two were attending vocational retraining after three years of occupational secondary school and one had finished secondary education. The remaining 10 youths were aged 19–21 years old; 2 of them were in secondary school and 8 were university students studying economics (4), social work (1), construction engineering (1), transportation science (1) and kinesiology (1). One boy had finished secondary school.

All of the participants had been placed as the result of inadequate parental care and all were living in the City of Zagreb where educational opportunities are the best in Croatia and, at least theoretically, accessible to all. Two of the children had moved for vocational retraining from a small town on the coast to Zagreb. The length of stay in out-of-home placement was 10 years on average.

Youth were informed about the research and invited to participate in focus groups by their care workers. The target population was all those living in independence units of children's homes and in the youth-community from an SOS children's village. All young people in the final years of secondary school and students were invited. Foster children can only be reached and invited to participate in research through care workers. So social workers did, inevitably, participate in the selection process, and the potential influence on data is unavoidable because we can assume that they invited the most cooperative children with whom they have the best contact. The young people chose whether or not to participate and also suggested the time of the focus group meeting.

Six focus groups, facilitated by the present authors, were held in three different locations. These were: a children's home independence unit (nine youth partici-pated), the youth-community from SOS children's village (nine youth participated) and in the Centre for Social Care with fostered children (13 youth participated). Issues raised in focus groups were: satisfaction with academic achievement and choice of school, experiences in school settings, support they have had or have at the moment and motivation for education. Discussions typically lasted for one hour, recorded on a digital voice recorder and subsequently transcribed verbatim.

Limitations of the Sample

There are some methodological issues that must be acknowledged. Since youth from children's homes were invited through their care workers and the focus group took place in the independence unit of the home where all the youth live together and see what is going on, it can be assumed that they participated because of social conformism. Their personal motivation might be weak but curiosity and the group setting influenced the decision to participate. Possibly as a result of this, in one focus group nine participants joined the session, which we experienced as a too large group for a fruitful discussion. Second, in that group several youth participated either passively or obstructed the discussion. That group was very challenging to moderate. Therefore, it might have been better to hold the focus group meeting in a neutral place outside the children's home facility. Fostered participants were invited through social workers and we can assume that they invited those youth with whom they had the best contacts. The youth who chose actively to participate in the research were interested in the topic, regularly attending school, so a question can be raised about the absence of low achievers and drop outs. The other reservation relates to the fact that, apart from one boy, all the foster youth were in kinship placements.

In the children's home and SOS children's village the young people knew one another. At the beginning of the group meetings the confidentiality issue was discussed and participants agreed not to talk about the content of discussion outside the group setting. The same discussion took place in focus groups with foster care youth who did not know one another. Two coders (both social workers and researchers) each separately performed analysis using qualitative content analysis on the same transcripts. After separate analysis results were considered jointly, some categories emerged for both researchers, and the categories that differed were discussed. The results have been summarised and will be presented in relation to three dimensions: youth perception of educational relevance, their experience of the educational process and factors that facilitate positive educational outcome.

Findings

Perception of Educational Relevance

All except two participants stated that education is important in the lives of children and youth. They talked about its relevance from two points of view—general relevance of education for children and youth, and personal educational relevance. Half of them pointed out that education is *equally important for all children,* no matter where or with whom they live, because education enables better life conditions and can improve employment possibilities:

> If you get a university degree people will look for you as a worker. You will have a bigger salary, better life . . .

The other half stated that education is *more important for children in public care* because they do not have a stable family base; they feel financial insecurity and pressure to be independent early, regardless of the type of placement:

> With whom and where are we going to live when we turn 18 years? We have to be independent, rent an apartment, pay the bills. For us education is more important so we can provide financial stability for ourselves.

> It is important, since we have no advantage at the start as other children have; for them it is not so important to get some kind of degree, but for us it will be easier if we have it, and it will be easier for us to become independent . . .

Young people see education as a path that can help them get out of their present situation, ensure future family life and normalisation. As one girl pointed out: 'school means a lot; it is the only thing that can help us'. With good education they can even help their biological family and avoid the possibility that their own children might get into the same situation as they have found themselves.

Two participants argued, on the contrary, that *education is not that important* because what matters is 'to pass through the hard school of life'. They questioned the value of education, having in mind economic crises, unemployment and business success stories of local celebrities with no formal higher education. Some also suspect that there is no way out of their situation, that their future is not bright with or without education:

> ...We see that successful people are those who lie and steal, things like that, not those with higher education. There is no use of education if you do not lie, steal, or swindle...

Not all took such a cynical view. Personal differences are more visible in the results that follow. The majority of respondents, students, grammar school youth from children's homes and most foster family youth have *high personal educational aspirations*. They have a clear area of interest, and had good grades in elementary and high school and plan to continue their education further:

> ...I was always a "nerd" interested in science, and I wanted to enrol in a good secondary school.

In contrast, more of the youth in residential care have *low personal aspirations for education*. They had low academic achievement in elementary school and are doing poorly now in secondary school, wishing to finish formal education as soon as possible. One boy said: 'I wanted to be free after secondary school'.

Experience in the Education Process

Another theme that was discussed in the focus groups is their experience in the education process. The majority of youth stated that they were actually quite satisfied with their educational achievement. They had already made some *educational choices* after elementary school. In the decision-making process about secondary school several factors were interwoven: personal wishes and aspirations, grades and influence from peers and adults. Those who had good grades and clear personal aspirations enrolled in the desired school. But for many youth the scope for choice was very narrow, due to low grades in elementary school. So they enrolled at the school with lowest entrance criteria and in courses of short duration, mainly occupational three-year programmes. There were eight young people with no personal aspirations who simply went 'with the flow'—followed their friends or accepted the advice of professionals from vocational guidance:

> I have no wish to enter work yet. I wish to achieve a higher level of knowledge. Of course, I want to be able to compete better (for jobs).

I finished elementary school and I did not know where to go. I had no desire to enter grammar school as after it I would have had to attend university, instead I wanted to be free after school...

During the last year of my elementary school I was sent to vocational guidance where they told me to attend vocational school for cosmetics, hair-dressing or pedicure and I decided to go for cosmetics. I did not want that, but I did not have any other choice.

Youth with no clear interests and those with low grades stated more frequently that they were not satisfied with the school they were attending, but some of them adjusted over time. As one girl said: 'Better anything than nothing'. Important were also some practical and organisational reasons, such as teaching available at different times of the day, the closeness of the school and employment possibilities promised by relatives. One boy explained: 'At that time, I was training for swimming and water polo. Only this school had afternoon shifts so I could practice in the morning, and that was it'.

Differences that emerged in youth experiences due to type of placement were connected with the influence and help from adults in the decision-making process concerning secondary education. Foster care youth stressed their independence in choosing a school. Children from residential care were influenced by their care workers and were regularly sent to vocational guidance. It was usually assumed that because of low grades in elementary school they would enrol in lower level vocational courses for routine or manual occupations:

...You play with children in the children's home and do not think about school. Each year some of the guys go to become plumbers so I went; but nobody asked me what I want to do and become in my life.

This boy pointed out that grades are very important, but personal aspirations should be taken much more seriously when deciding about secondary school. If the child in care has low grades they automatically go to vocational school, no matter what their personal interests or employment aspirations might be. If the child has good grades, he or she can try to enrol in grammar school, but that seems to be rare. An extreme example is the experience of one girl who was enrolled in secondary school by her care workers without her knowing anything about it at all. She stresses that she is very unhappy in her school: 'I would not go to that school at all, it is something that I do not like'.

In accordance with their prevailing belief that education is important, most of the youth reported that they would like to continue education at university. But, for the majority this is not a realistic possibility due to their grades and type of secondary school attended.

They talked about *circumstances that promote and those that impede* their education. Facilitating circumstances are related to their schools, primarily with teachers who are willing to help and to be cooperative, with pupils, and with subjects that they like and can learn without too much effort. Relationships with friends and care workers (for youth in residential care) also help them in their education. Living conditions are important for them as well, especially conditions conducive to study, such as having their own room. Youth from residential care pointed to the usefulness of extra-curricular activities that were organised by the home (sport activities) while youth in foster families perceive summer camps and other workshops that are organised for them as a good way to make friends and socialise. Scholarships are very important for students:

> It is much easier when you know you have some additional financial support (scholarship) which is more generous than pocket money from the children's home.

Some youth perceived difficult school subjects, old-fashioned authoritarian teachers and poor relationships with peers as circumstances that impede their education. Besides school-oriented situations, youth mention personal factors, such as more interest in other things and lack of support as impeding circumstances. Also, they pointed to the current economic crisis and lower employment possibilities as discouraging factors. As shown earlier, they feel the pressure to become independent after secondary school or university education since they have to leave care without a secure family base. Therefore, they perceive employment possibilities as very important, but fear it will be hard for them to find jobs due to the economic climate and they would like more support in that regard:

> After secondary school we do not have secure employment which bothers me. Now we have to pass graduation exams. Learn different, sometimes unnecessary things to pass it and maybe enrol at university, but at the end I will finish at the unemployment office.

When asked about support in the educational process, the young people mainly mentioned friends or said they had nobody, saying that they could depend only on themselves. Only a few of them keep in contact with someone outside of their placements, like parents, siblings or other relatives. When we asked them about relationships with social workers only a few stated that they have contact with them. Some of them did not even know who their social worker was. Most of them lack close stable relationships, while the position of some can be regarded as highly isolated and lonely.

Some of the youth experienced a *differentiated approach to in-care children* in schools. They report that teachers have lower expectations of them and apply lower standards: 'Teachers are complaisant, they understand our situation, they let us pass easily'. Residential care workers often beg teachers to give the child a good enough mark. Curiosity and sometimes pity from their peers as well as teachers are also part of the school experience of children in care.

In relation to the type of placement we found another difference in youth educational experience. Children in residential care experienced greater stigmatisation.

Their placement in a children's home is often confused with placement in a correctional institution, so the initial reaction of peers and, even more often of teachers and other school employees, is negative: '...until they get to know us better':

> When you say you live in a children's home, everybody is thinking of correctional institutions, they say-you make problems, stay away from me...

> In the locker room two mobile phones went missing and immediately they assumed it was me because I am from a children's home. It turned out that it was a girl from a rich family.

Foster youth often claimed that there were no differences in attitudes towards them and other children, but they often hide their life situation from school. They said that only class teachers and a few very best friends know their background and: 'I do not talk about it, there is no need'. Students who lived in independence units of children's homes also stressed that they do not talk about that because at university it is not relevant: 'What matters is how you succeed in your studies'.

Facilitation of Positive Educational Outcomes

Insights on this dimension were provided by a group of higher achievers—college students and grammar school pupils regardless of type of placement. They highlighted their own *personal strength and self-efficacy* as important predictors of educational outcome. What they stressed as their advantages were individual commitment to school, faith in their personal capacities and a good image of themselves as being strong. They explained their academic successes by these characteristics, which differentiate them from their peers in public care:

> I had the opportunity and I realised I have to finish school. I was always more diligent and learned more than my peers. In my opinion it has nothing to do either with placement or family, I simply wanted to be better.

> I made myself learn. I do not know about the others. It depends on the person.

Youth perceive *financial support* as the most significant condition that can influence their educational possibilities. What they perceive as minimum requirements are scholarships for living expenses and fees, secure accommodation, free books and transportation.

Higher achievers from residential care pointed out the importance of *relationship with the professionals*. Particular professionals were described as very engaged, patient, warm, those who spotted their possibilities and provided them with support and motivation to learn and aspire for more. They stress that care workers in general should pay more attention to all children with good grades, who are not 'troublemakers', and who could achieve more with adequate support:

> I was lucky to come to the best care worker in the children's home. She worked equally with everybody and through discussion and encouragement urged us to fulfil our potential . . . the relationship with her was easy and friendly.

Some, although very few, told of good contact with social workers who were helpful, interested and reachable when needed:

> My (social worker) really cares about me. For the last seven years, from the day I entered the children's home, she has provided everything I need. She gives me within a single day [i.e. without delay] any approval or permission I ask for, e.g. for a school excursion.

Other youth who have had no contact or less helpful dealings with social workers have questioned that relationship and given us some insights in terms of practical advice. They state the importance of keeping promises, not lying about length of placement and recommend that social workers should keep in regular contact with the child. Furthermore, they suggest that social workers should pay more attention to individual cases, carefully assess the situation of the child, be better informed themselves and give more information about all the rights and options available to children in public care regarding education.

Does Care Improve or Diminish Educational Opportunities?

A new insight in this study relates to current educational possibilities as compared to those offered by their biological family. Despite the shortcomings identified earlier, most of our respondents considered that their opportunities would be far less if they had remained with their birth families. The majority of youth stated that they would have finished elementary school at best, or maybe some secondary school but few would even think about university. Students and some secondary school pupils pointed out that they are already more educated than their parents. It seems that these youth see placement in public care as offering some improvement to their life chances.

Discussion

The goal of this research has been to obtain a user's perspective of educational relevance through the experiences of youth in public care in Croatia. The results showed that youth consider education as important, but their personal aspirations, strengths and potentials differ. Most youth perceive education as being of high importance because it improves employment possibilities and enhances overall life chances. Some of the youth think that education is even more important for those in public care, because they know that they have to become economically independent at an early age and they see education as a way to get qualifications that can ensure better employment opportunities. Leaving the care system, these young people have to deal with adult issues at once—leaving a familiar place, finding a new home, finding a job, setting up a family, pursuing further educational opportunities, or coping with failure in all these areas without the possibility of going back into the care system in difficult times, such as becoming unemployed. We can say that the youth in our sample felt quite alone, with no financial support and pressured by the care system to be independent because they cannot stay in public care after turning 18, with the exception of continuing education. At the same time support by birth families is poor or absent, family connections are usually problematic so youth lack the financial, practical and emotional support needed through this life stage. As Mike Stein has pointed out that in relation to young people leaving care in the UK, their journey to adulthood is both accelerated and compressed (Stein, 2006, p. 274). It is a very different experience from that of the majority of their peers.

Although their school grades and the fact that most attend occupational secondary schools show that their educational attainment is below average, the young people themselves are generally satisfied with their performance and perceive that their educational possibilities are better than if they had stayed with their own parents. Therefore, it could be said that the purpose of child welfare intervention, at least in terms of education and assuring better life chances, has been fulfilled from the youths' perspective. This is in contrast to findings from some other countries, such as Sweden and England (Jackson, 2000; Vinnerljung et al., 2005; Berridge, 2007), that compensatory effects of care on education are at best neutral. Similar to our findings, Gallagher et al. (2004) showed that residential care can be a positive environment for educational achievement, especially if children are given a sense of the value of education, clear expectations about it, and are provided with a learning culture and good support. Many of our respondents wish for better educational opportunities and obviously see the importance of education for social inclusion (in the form of good employment and normal living conditions), but it is out of reach for most of them due to low grades and inadequate secondary schools that are not preparing them sufficiently for higher levels of education.

Our findings are supportive of so-called 'resilience-led practice' (Daniel, 2003). We have found from the testimony of young people in our study as well as our own practice experience that what favours resilience and better educational attainment is having a secure base, self-esteem and self-efficacy, and adults who have provided consistent support. Those youth with sufficient educational skills, grades and high aspirations emphasise their personal capacities and strengths that help them in the educational process. They have also had experience of good stable relationships with at least one professional who supported and motivated them to aspire for more and to study harder.

Many international authors stress the importance of encouragement and positive influences from carers and significant others outside their placement regarding higher educational outcomes for children in public care (Martin & Jackson, 2002; Harker et al., 2004). Our youth strongly rely only on themselves or keep in mind a good care worker from earlier years. In most cases they did not mention their parents, relatives, teachers or social workers as of any importance to their education. Contrary to

Dearden's (2004) findings that support givers were teachers, social workers, family members and foster carers but that residential carers were unhelpful, in our research residential care workers were most likely to be supportive, at least to high achievers. But obviously, many Croatian youth in care are not living in an educationally rich environment, as defined by Connelly *et al.* (2003), and are missing a range of facilities and professional support that they require and wish for.

A differentiated approach towards youth in-care reported by participants is in agreement with many other studies. Negative stereotypes and labelling by teachers and others, including social workers, have been found to be major obstacles to success in school settings. Children and young people in public care are regarded as delinquents not interested in school or not having the potential for academic success (Francis, 2000; Jackson & Sachdev, 2001; Martin & Jackson, 2002). The fact that young people who are looked after have low attainments confirms the low expectations, which have typically been held by many professionals, without taking account of the conditions that depress their school performance (Connelly & Chakrabarti, 2008). Assumptions that they are in care because of their own fault and behavioural disorders and not as a result of family circumstances, further reduce their self-esteem, already low because of experiences of abuse, abandonment and rejection (Schofield *et al.*, 2000).

In considering the future prospects for the youth who took part in our focus groups we found the threefold classification proposed by Stein was helpful (Stein, 2006). Our results showed that a majority of our participants are likely to be *moving on*—being the youth whose resilience has been improved by care experiences, who had stable placements and secure attachments, who achieved some educational success and are hoping to find a job they like and have a family like other 'normal' people. Other youth participating in the study could be classified as *survivors*—those who see themselves as self-reliant and more grown-up than their peers, valuing their unfavourable life experiences as important 'school of life'. However, compared with the first group, they will leave care younger, with fewer qualifications and have lower paid jobs and more problems, though hopefully keeping a sense of independence. In our sample we had almost no youth in the third group, which Stein describes as *victims*—those who had the most damaging pre-care experiences and continued to suffer in care, often changing placements, having disrupted relationships and education. This is the group in greatest danger of social exclusion. After leaving care they are often unemployed, homeless, lonely, isolated, and have mental health problems with no aftercare support. The reason why this group did not appear in our research is probably explained by the way the participants were recruited, as explained earlier. It can be assumed that either they did not want to participate or we failed to reach them. It is very important for future research that this group of in-care youth should be approached also, since they have the greatest risk of future life failures.

Despite these methodological issues and some historical and professional differences from other countries, Croatian research on child welfare and the results presented here on care leavers provide some indication of how educational and overall well-being of in-care children and youth could be enhanced.

To conclude, a comprehensive approach to educational issues is necessary, aiming to improve life opportunities of youth in public care and to provide a better and more gradual transition to an out-of-care future. It should contain a far stronger engagement of social – and care workers in finding ways to enhance young people's personal strengths and objective opportunities. Every in-care child's perspective and motives should be explored, and aspiration of any kind supported. We strongly agree with Pecora *et al.* (2006) on the importance of orientating teachers and schools to be aware of in-care issues, providing youth and their caregivers with detailed information on further educational possibilities, and raising awareness and outreach of these possibilities for them. Providing financial and other practical support and securing employment possibilities would give youth a sense of basic security. Our work has shown that detailed research on the attitudes and practice of social work professionals must be undertaken and new possibilities for those leaving care must be devised and implemented, following models from some other countries, such as needs assessment and pathway planning, integrated school and care plans, independent living programs, ongoing support for those in post-compulsory education and mentoring (Montgomery *et al.*, 2006; Osterling & Hines, 2006; Wade & Dixon, 2006). But it must not be forgotten that improving educational opportunities for children in care equally concerns their present developmental needs as well as their future opportunities.

References

Ajduković, M. (2004) 'Approaches to the care of children without adequate parental care in Europe', *Journal of Social Policy*, vol. 11, no. 3–4, pp. 299–220 (in Croatian).

Ajduković, M. (2008) 'Early interventions and other community based interventions as a support to families in risk?', in *The Children's Right to Live in a Family*, eds M. Ajdukoviá & T. Radočaj, Unicef-Office for Croatia, Zagreb, pp. 57–76 (in Croatian).

Ajduković, M. & Sladović Franz, B. (2005) 'Behavioral and emotional problems of children by type of out-of-home care in Croatia', *International Journal of Social Welfare*, vol. 14, pp. 163–175.

Berridge, D. (2007) 'Theory and explanation in child welfare: education and looked after children', *Child and Family Social Work*, vol. 12, no. 1, pp. 1–10.

Connelly, G. (2003) 'Developing quality indicators for learning with care', *Scottish Journal of Residential Child Care*, vol. 2, no. 2, pp. 69–78.

Connelly, G. & Chakrabarti, M. (2008) 'Improving the educational experience of children and young people in public care: a Scottish perspective', *International Journal of Inclusive Education*, vol. 12, no. 4, pp. 347–361.

Daniel, B. (2003) 'The value of resilience as a concept for practice in residential settings', *Scottish Journal of Residential Child Care*, vol. 2, no. 1, pp. 6–16.

Dearden, J. (2004) 'Resilience: a study of risk and protective factors from the perspective of young people with experience of local authority care', *Support for Learning*, vol. 19, no. 4, pp. 187–193.

Dent, R. J. & Cameron, S. (2003) 'Developing resilience in children who are in public care: the educational psychology perspective', *Educational Psychology in Practice*, vol. 19, no. 1, pp. 3–19.

Flick, U., von Kardorff, E. & Steinke, I. (2004) *A Companion to Qualitative Research*, Sage, London.

Francis, J. (2000) 'Investing in children's futures: enhancing the educational arrangements of "looked after" children and young people', *Child and Family Social Work*, vol. 5, pp. 23–33.

Gallagher, B., Brannan, C., Jones, R. & Westwood, S. (2004) 'Good practice in the education of children in residential care', *British Journal of Social Work*, vol. 34, no. 8, pp. 1133–1160.

Gudbrandsson, B. (2003) *Children at Risk and in Care*, Council of Europe, Social Cohesion Social Policy Department, Strasbourg.

Harker, R., Dobel-Ober, D., Akhurts, S. & Sinclair, R. (2004) 'Who takes care of education 18 months on? A follow-up study of looked after children's perception of support for educational progress', *Child and Family Social Work*, vol. 9, pp. 273–284.

Jackson, S. (2000) 'Promoting the educational achievement of looked-after children', in *Combating Educational Disadvantage: Meeting the Needs of Vulnerable Children*, ed. T. Cox, Falmer Press, London, pp. 65–80.

Jackson, S. (2007) 'Care leavers, exclusion and access to higher education', in *Multiprofessional Hanbook of Social Exclusion*, eds D. Abrams, J. Christian & D. Gordon, Chichester, Wiley, pp. 115–136.

Jackson, S. & Sachdev, D. (2001) *Better Education, Better Futures: Research, Practice and the Views of Young People in Care*, Barnardo's, Ilford.

Jackson, S. & Cameron, C. (2012) *Final Report of the YiPPEE Project WP 12 – Young People from a Public Care Background: Pathways to Further and Higher Education in Five European Countries*, Thomas Coram Research Unit, Insitute of Education, University of London, [Online] Available at: http://tcru.ioe.ac.uk/yippee/Portals/1/Final%20Report%20of%20the%20YiPPEE%20Project%20-%20WP12%20Mar11.pdf

Korintus, M., Racz, A. & Czak, R. (2010) *Young People in Public Care: Pathways to Education in Europe (YiPPEE) Hungary National Report*, [Online] Available at: http://tcru.ioe.ac.uk/yippee

Kregar Orešković, K. & Rajhvajn, L. (2007) 'Characteristic of life and psychosocial needs of boys and girls growing up in foster families', *Child and Society*, vol. 9, no. 1, pp. 63–88 (in Croatian).

Martin, P. Y. & Jackson, S. (2002) 'Educational success for children in public care: advice from a group of high achievers', *Child and Family Social Work*, vol. 7, pp. 121–130.

Ministry of Health and Social Welfare Croatia. (2010) *Statistical Report*, Ministry of Health and Social Welfare, Zagreb.

Montgomery, P., Donkoh, C. & Underhill, K. (2006) 'Independent living programs for young people leaving the care system: the state of evidence', *Children and Youth Services Review*, vol. 28, pp. 1435–1448.

Ministry of Family, Veteran's Affairs and Intergenerational Solidarity. (2006) *National Activity Plan for Children's Rights and Interests 2006–2012*, Council for Children, Zagreb.

Osterling, K. & Hines, A. (2006) 'Mentoring adolescent foster youth: promoting resilience during developmental transitions', *Child and Family Social Work*, vol. 11, pp. 242–253.

Pecora, J. P., Williams, J., Kessler, R. C., Hiripi, E., O'Brien, K., Emerson, J., Herrick, M. A. & Torres, D. (2006) 'Assessing the educational achievements of adults who were formerly placed in family foster care', *Child and Family Social Work*, vol. 11, pp. 220–231.

Schofield, G., Beek, M., Sargent, K. & Thoburn, J. (2000) *Growing Up in Foster Care*, BAAF, London.

Sladović Franz, B. (2004) 'Predictors of behavioural and emotional problems of children placed in children's homes in Croatia', *Child and Family Social Work*, vol. 9, pp. 265–271.

Stein, M. (2006) 'Research review: young people leaving care', *Child and Family Social Work*, vol. 11, pp. 273–279.

Vinnerljung, B., Öman, M. & Gunnarson, T. (2005) 'Educational attainments of former child welfare clients – a Swedish national cohort study', *International Journal of Social Welfare*, vol. 15, pp. 265–276.

Wade, J. & Dixon, J. (2006) 'Making a home, finding a job: investigating early housing and employment outcomes for young people leaving care', *Child and Family Social Work*, vol. 11, pp. 199–208.

Index

Note: Page numbers in *italics* represent tables
Page numbers in **bold** represent figures
Page numbers followed by 'n' refer to notes